Creative Sole

A Chinese Reflexology Coloring Book for Adults to Relax and Get Your Qi Flowing

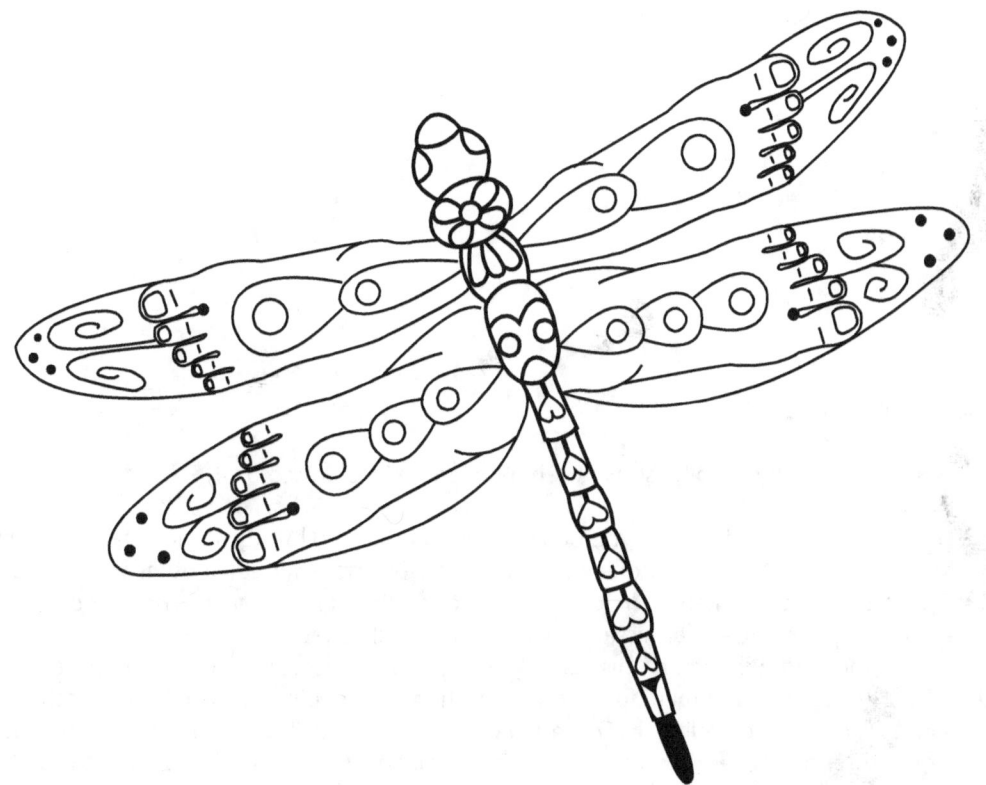

Holly Tse

ISBN: 9781441403490
1st edition, December 2019

Introduction

Welcome to the world of creative soles, the first ever Chinese Reflexology adult coloring book! You are clearly a creative soul with a passion for healing.

One of the best ways to improve your health and vitality is to get your qi flowing. Qi is the life force energy that flows through energy meridians in your body—similar to how blood flows through your veins and arteries. When qi is flowing smoothly and abundantly, your body is in a state of health. But when this energy becomes depleted or blocked, that's when physical issues can arise.

Chinese Reflexology is an ancient healing art based on the principles of Traditional Chinese Medicine. Reflexology points on your feet connect with the body's energy meridians and also correlate to different parts of the body. By massaging these points, you can improve the flow of qi through the meridians.

This coloring book presents a selection of Chinese Reflexology points and some interesting points (bad pun intended) related to the points. To learn how to massage your feet, I would recommend my book, Sole Guidance. It contains information on how to properly practice Chinese Reflexology, but it's almost 70,000 words in length!

Since too much thinking can interfere with the flow of qi, I chose not to overload this coloring book with too much information as it would take away from the fun and "flowy" experience of simply coloring. My intention for Creative Sole is to get your qi flowing through relaxation, playfulness and creativity.

Have FUN coloring!

Holly

P.S. If you'd like to learn more about Chinese Reflexology, check out the back of this coloring book for more ways to learn.

CHINESE REFLEXOLOGY 1❂1

萬 壽 無 疆

Holly Tse

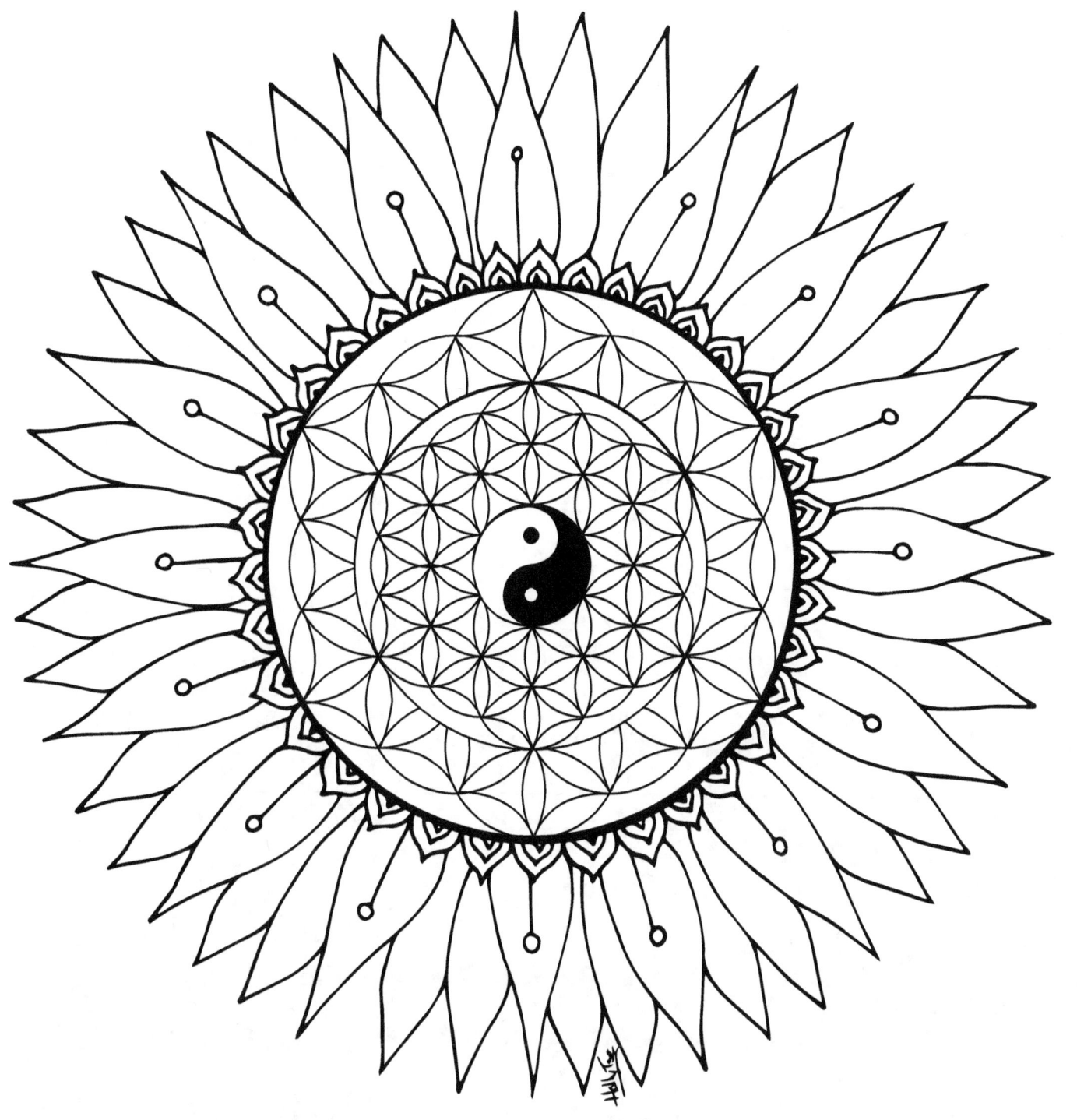

Yin and Yang

Yin represents female, dark, cold, night, and earth.
In the body, yin elements are blood, fluids, and anatomy.
Yang represents male, light, heat, day, and sun. In the body, yang
elements are energy, processes, and physiology.

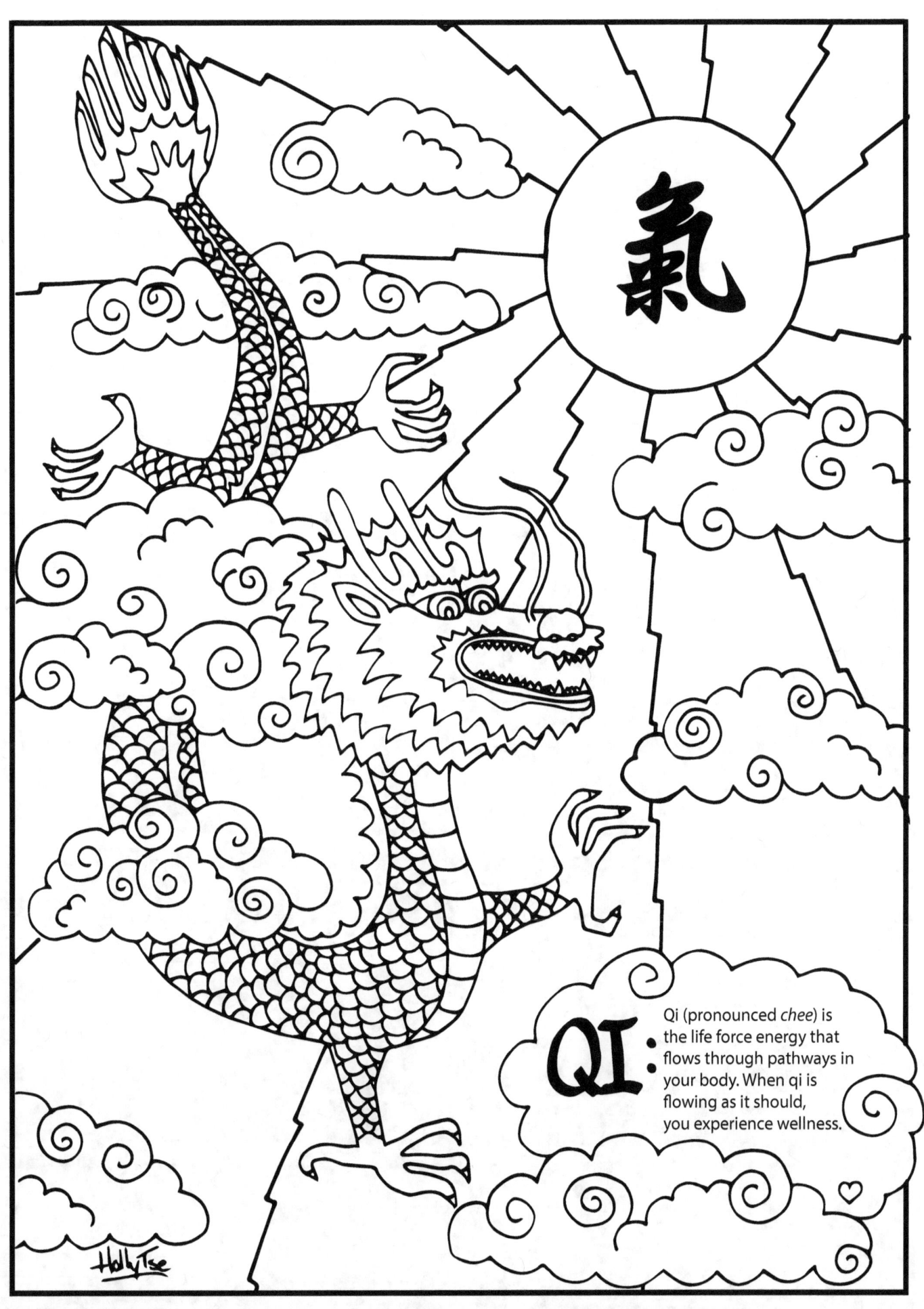

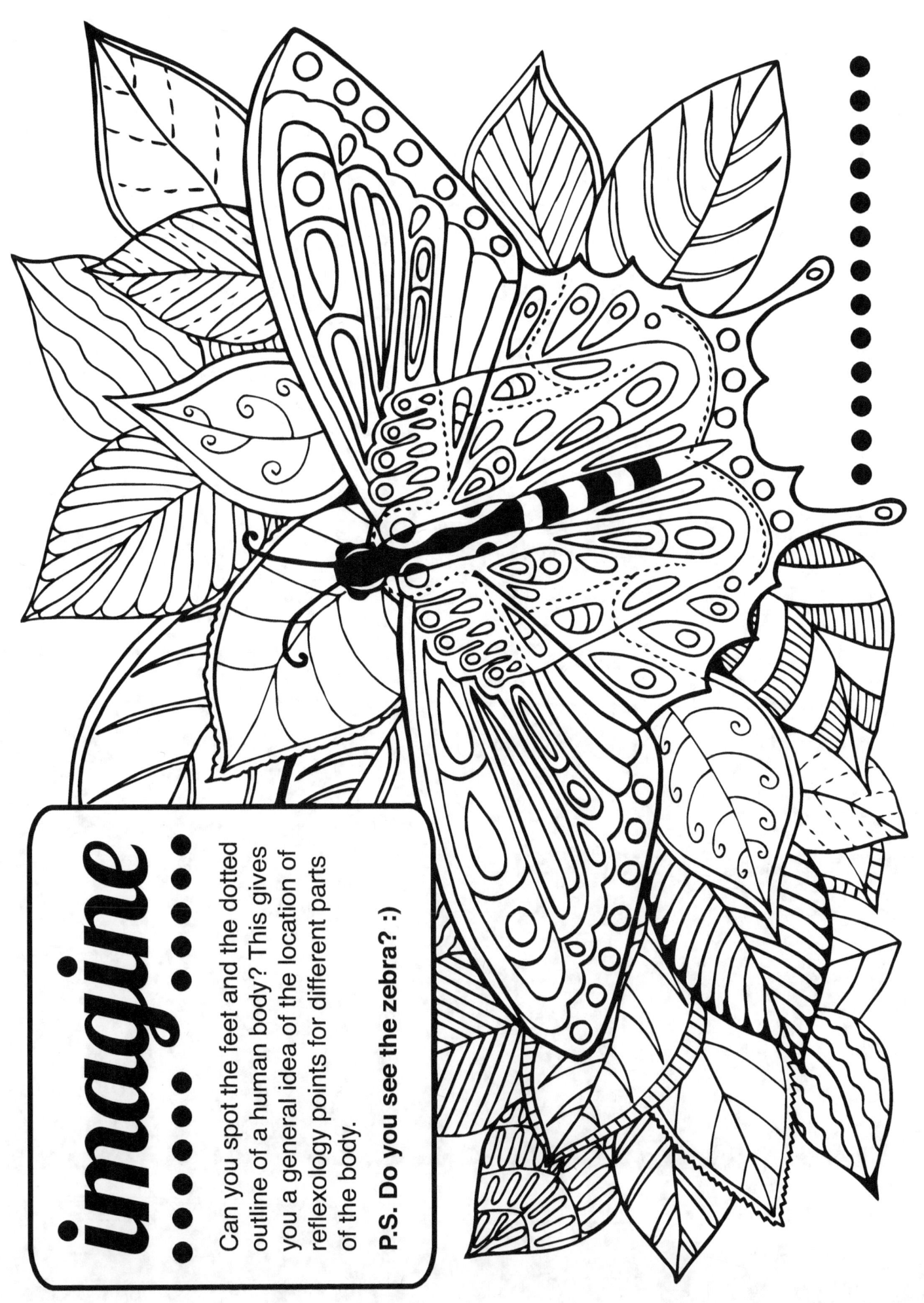

imagine

Can you spot the feet and the dotted outline of a human body? This gives you a general idea of the location of reflexology points for different parts of the body.

P.S. Do you see the zebra? :)

CHINESE REFLEXOLOGY CHARTS

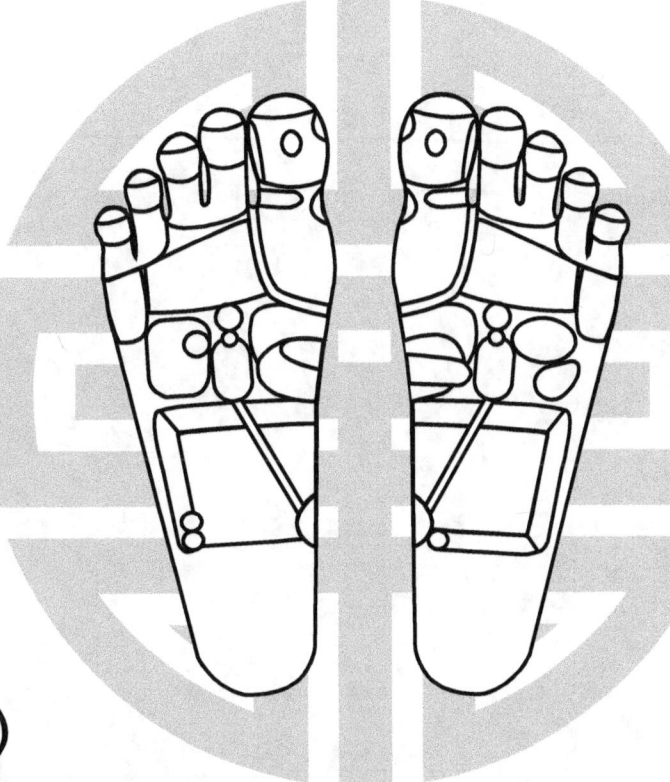

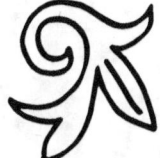

LEFT SOLE

Create your own color key for the Chinese Reflexology points on the left sole. Learn more at www.ChineseFootReflexology.com.

- ☐ 1. Sinus
- ☐ 2. Nose
- ☐ 3. Brain
- ☐ 4. Pituitary
- ☐ 5. Temporal Area
- ☐ 6. Parathyroid
- ☐ 7. Neck
- ☐ 8. Eye
- ☐ 9. Ear
- ☐ 10. Thyroid
- ☐ 11. Lung
- ☐ 12. Shoulder
- ☐ 13. Stomach
- ☐ 14. Duodenum

- ☐ 15. Pancreas
- ☐ 16. Solar Plexus
- ☐ 17. Adrenal
- ☐ 18. Kidney
- ☐ 19. Heart
- ☐ 20. Spleen
- ☐ 21. Transverse Colon
- ☐ 22. Ureter Tube
- ☐ 23. Small Intestine
- ☐ 24. Descending Colon
- ☐ 25. Bladder
- ☐ 26. Anus/Rectum
- ☐ 27. Sigmoid Colon

RIGHT SOLE

Create your own color key for the Chinese Reflexology points on the right sole. Learn more at www.ChineseFootReflexology.com.

- [ ] 1. Sinus
- [ ] 2. Nose
- [ ] 3. Brain
- [ ] 4. Pituitary
- [ ] 5. Temporal Area
- [ ] 6. Parathyroid
- [ ] 7. Neck
- [ ] 8. Eye
- [ ] 9. Ear
- [ ] 10. Thyroid
- [ ] 11. Lung
- [ ] 12. Shoulder
- [ ] 13. Stomach
- [ ] 14. Duodenum

- [ ] 15. Pancreas
- [ ] 16. Solar Plexus
- [ ] 17. Adrenal
- [ ] 18. Kidney
- [ ] 19. Liver
- [ ] 20. Gall Bladder
- [ ] 21. Transverse Colon
- [ ] 22. Ureter Tube
- [ ] 23. Small Intestine
- [ ] 24. Ascending Colon
- [ ] 25. Bladder
- [ ] 26. Ileocecal Valve
- [ ] 27. Appendix

INSIDE EDGE

Create your own color key. For the inside edge, the point locations are the same for both feet. Learn more at www.ChineseFootReflexology.com.

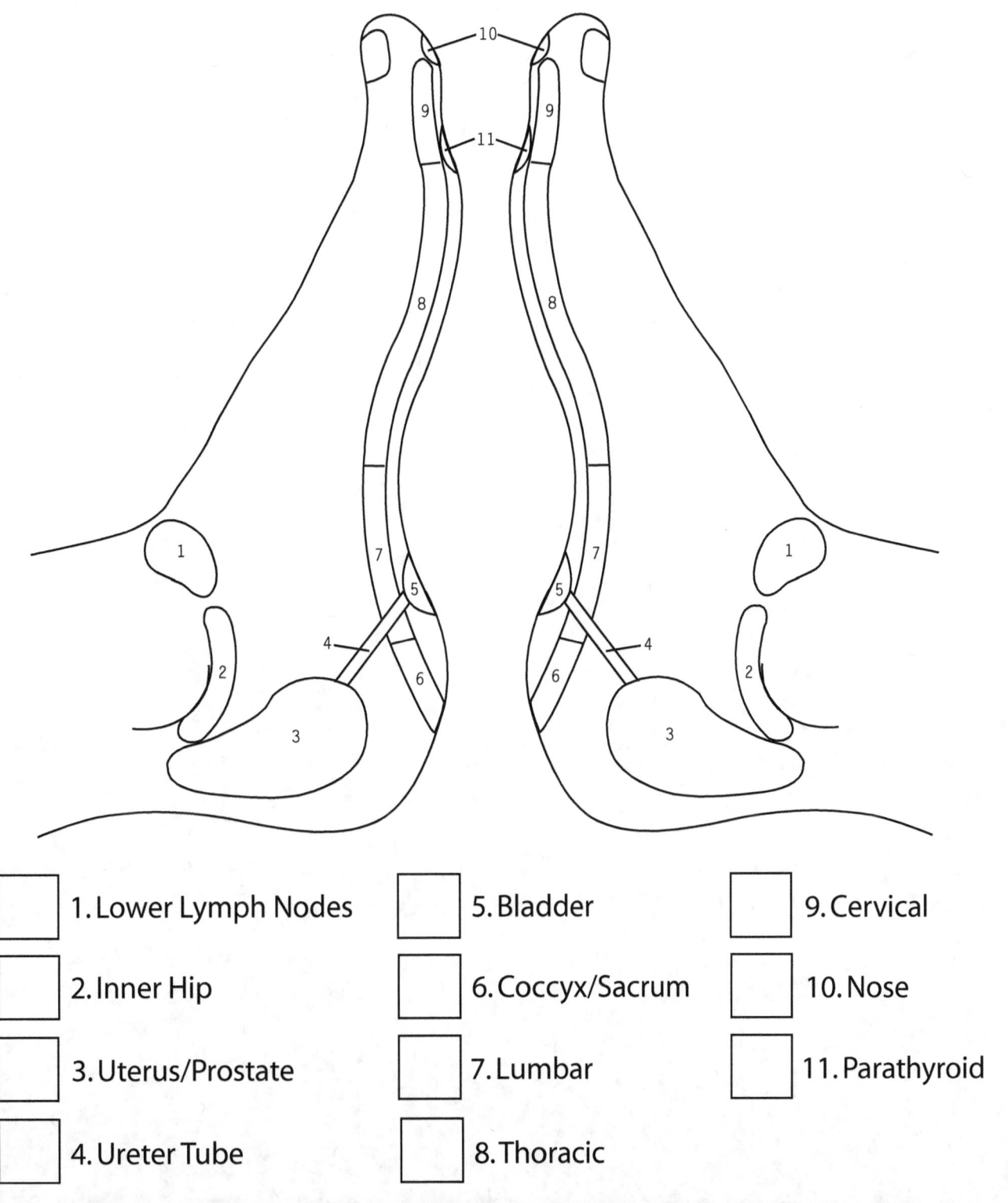

☐ 1. Lower Lymph Nodes

☐ 2. Inner Hip

☐ 3. Uterus/Prostate

☐ 4. Ureter Tube

☐ 5. Bladder

☐ 6. Coccyx/Sacrum

☐ 7. Lumbar

☐ 8. Thoracic

☐ 9. Cervical

☐ 10. Nose

☐ 11. Parathyroid

OUTSIDE EDGE

Create your own color key. For the outside edge, the point locations are the same for both feet. Learn more at www.ChineseFootReflexology.com.

1. Temporal Area

2. Shoulder

3. Knee

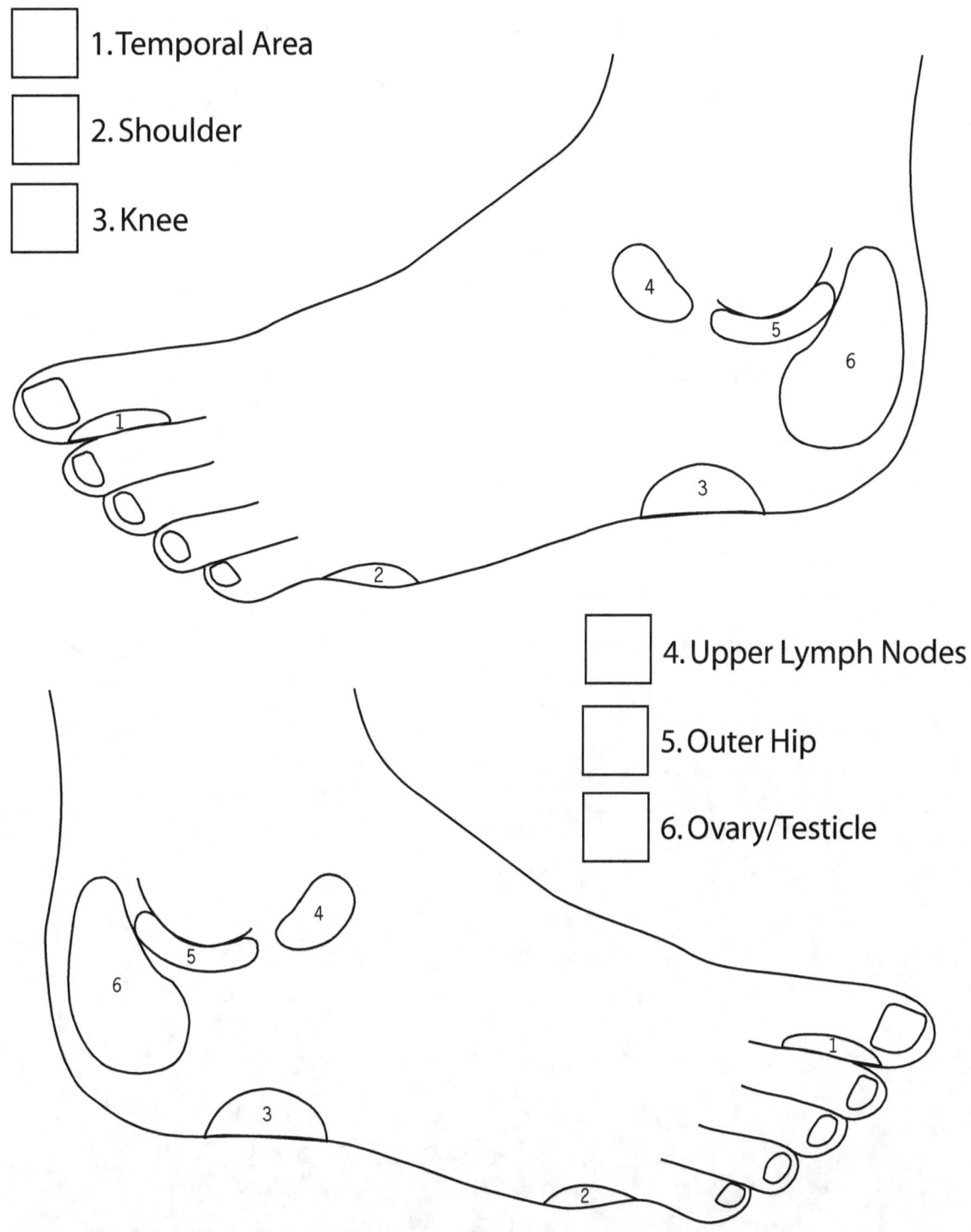

4. Upper Lymph Nodes

5. Outer Hip

6. Ovary/Testicle

OUTSIDE EDGE

TOP OF FOOT

Create your own color key. For the top, the point locations are the same for both feet. Learn more at www.ChineseFootReflexology.com.

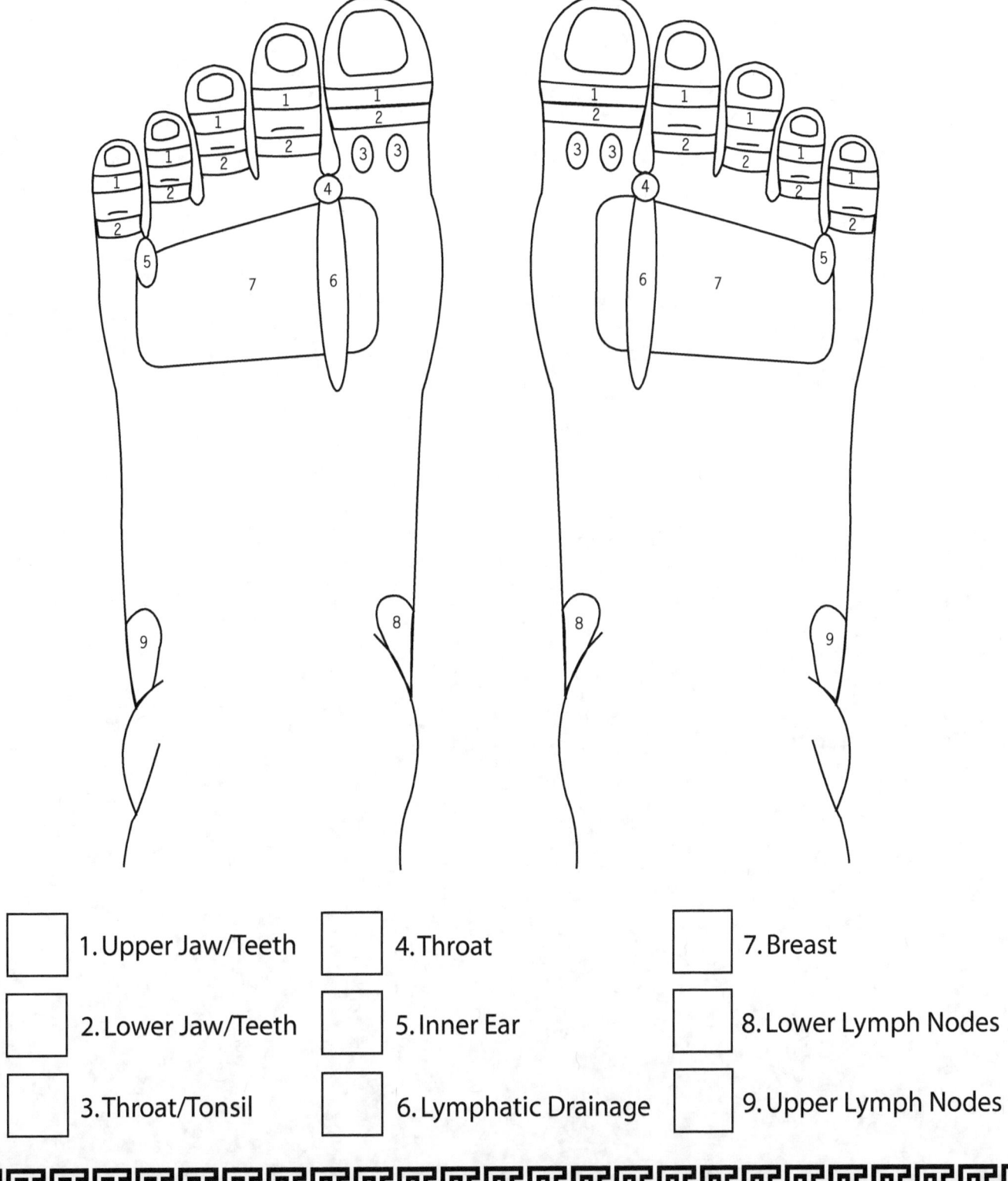

☐	1. Upper Jaw/Teeth	☐	4. Throat	☐	7. Breast
☐	2. Lower Jaw/Teeth	☐	5. Inner Ear	☐	8. Lower Lymph Nodes
☐	3. Throat/Tonsil	☐	6. Lymphatic Drainage	☐	9. Upper Lymph Nodes

Kidney

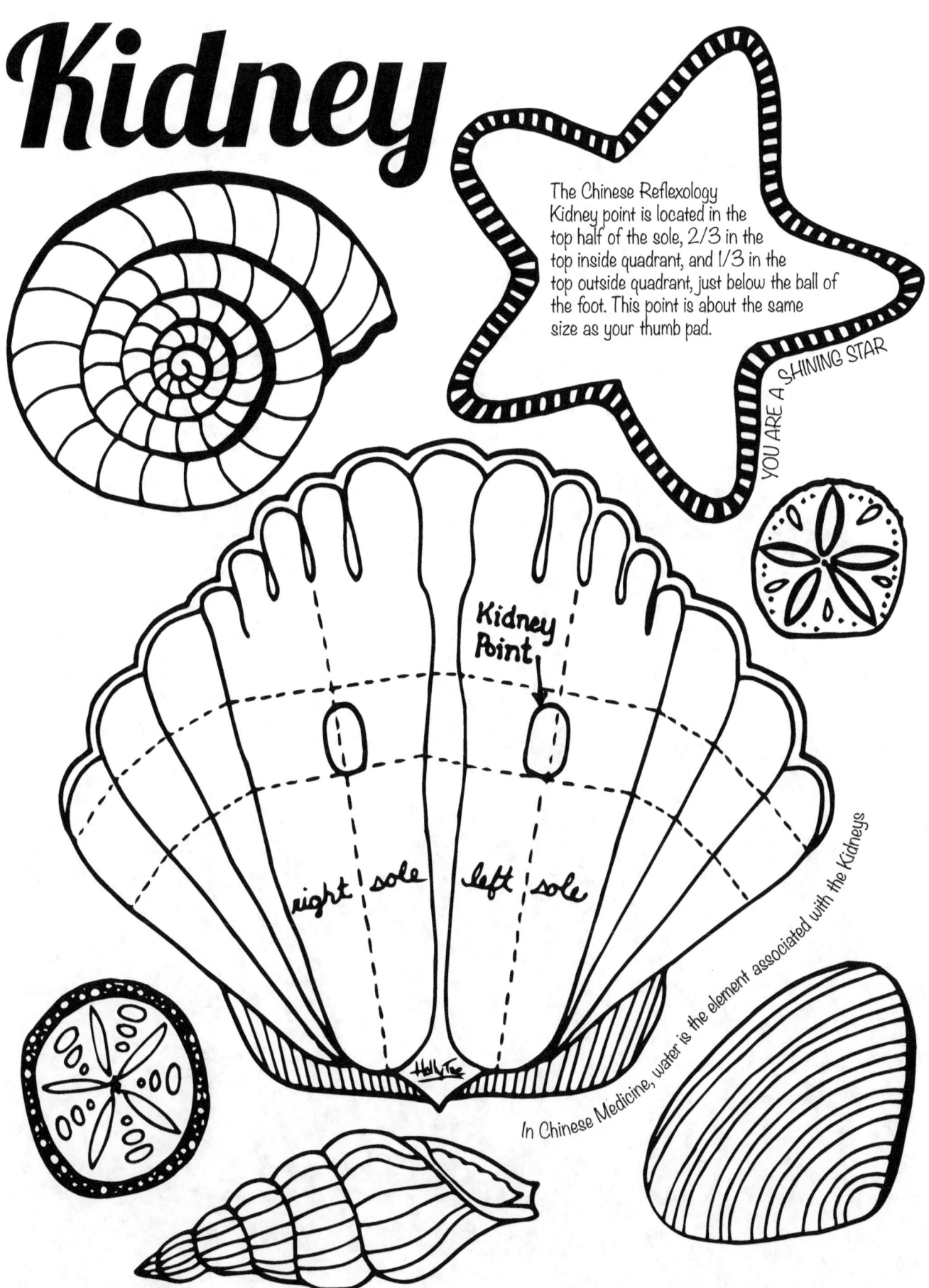

The Chinese Reflexology Kidney point is located in the top half of the sole, 2/3 in the top inside quadrant, and 1/3 in the top outside quadrant, just below the ball of the foot. This point is about the same size as your thumb pad.

YOU ARE A SHINING STAR

Kidney Point

right sole   left sole

In Chinese Medicine, water is the element associated with the Kidneys

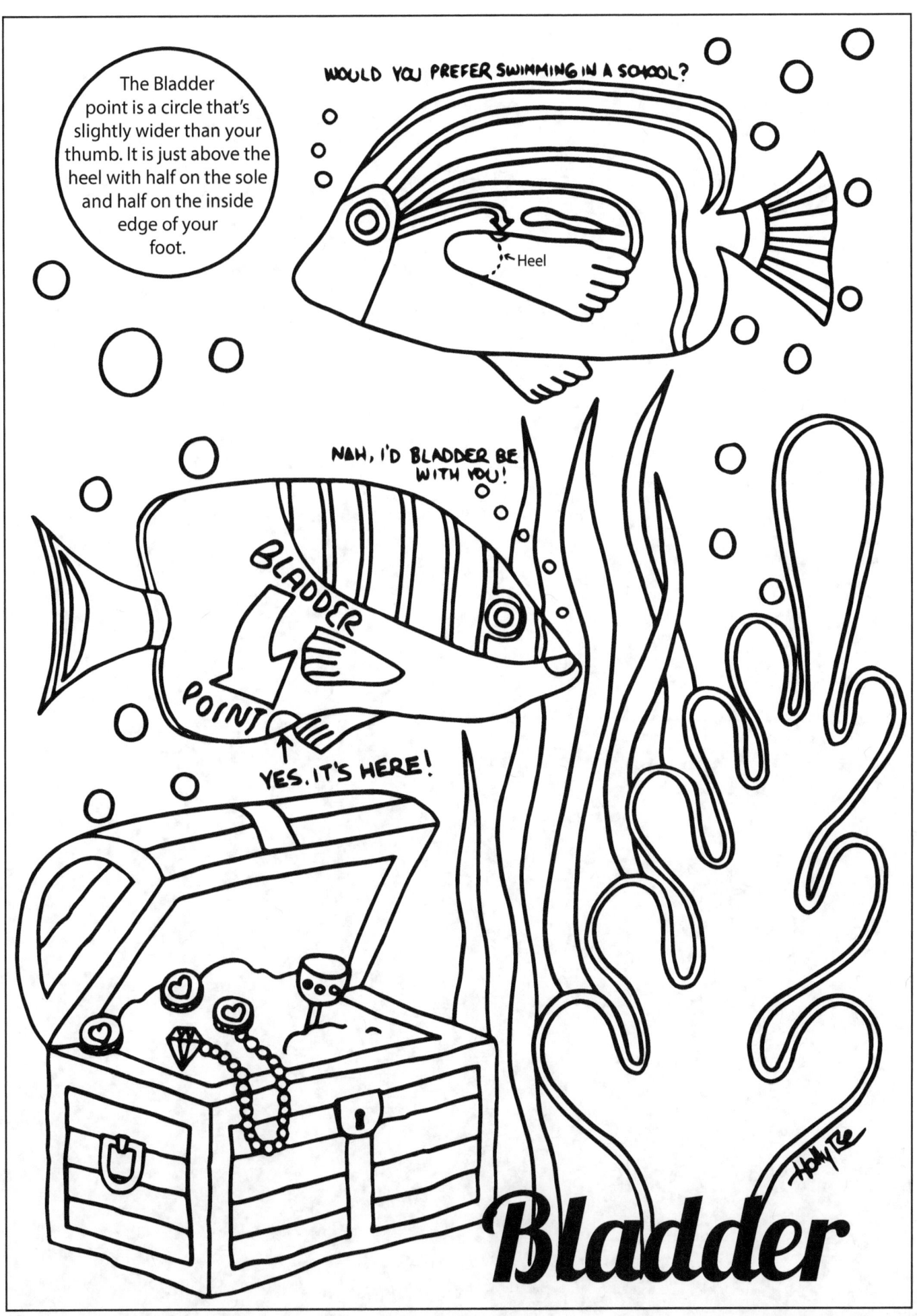

LYMPHATIC DRAINAGE

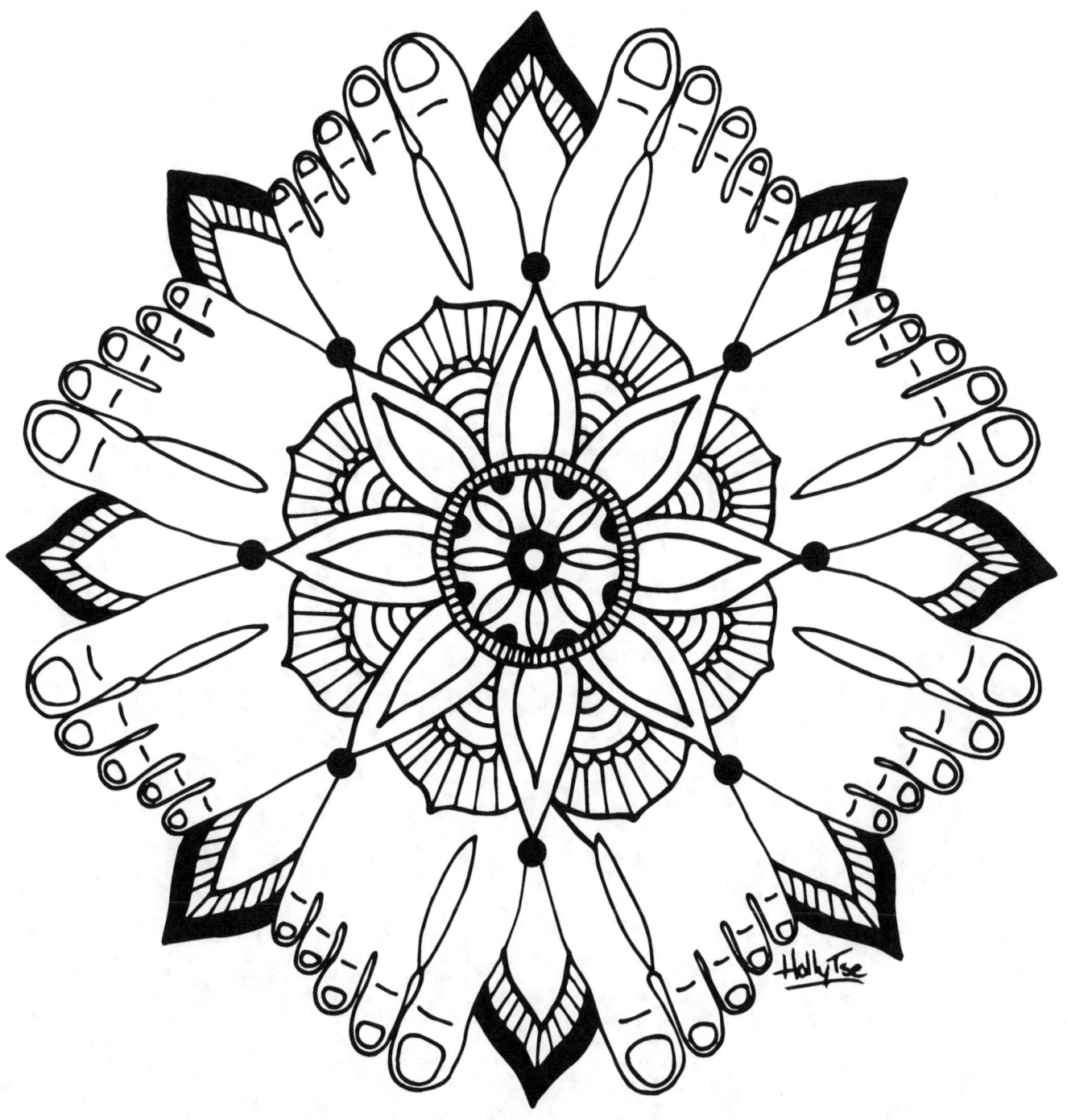

The Chinese Reflexology lymphatic drainage point is located on the tops of both feet. It's in the webbing between the big toe and second toe, from the base of the toes to the point of the V formed where the bones meet each other.

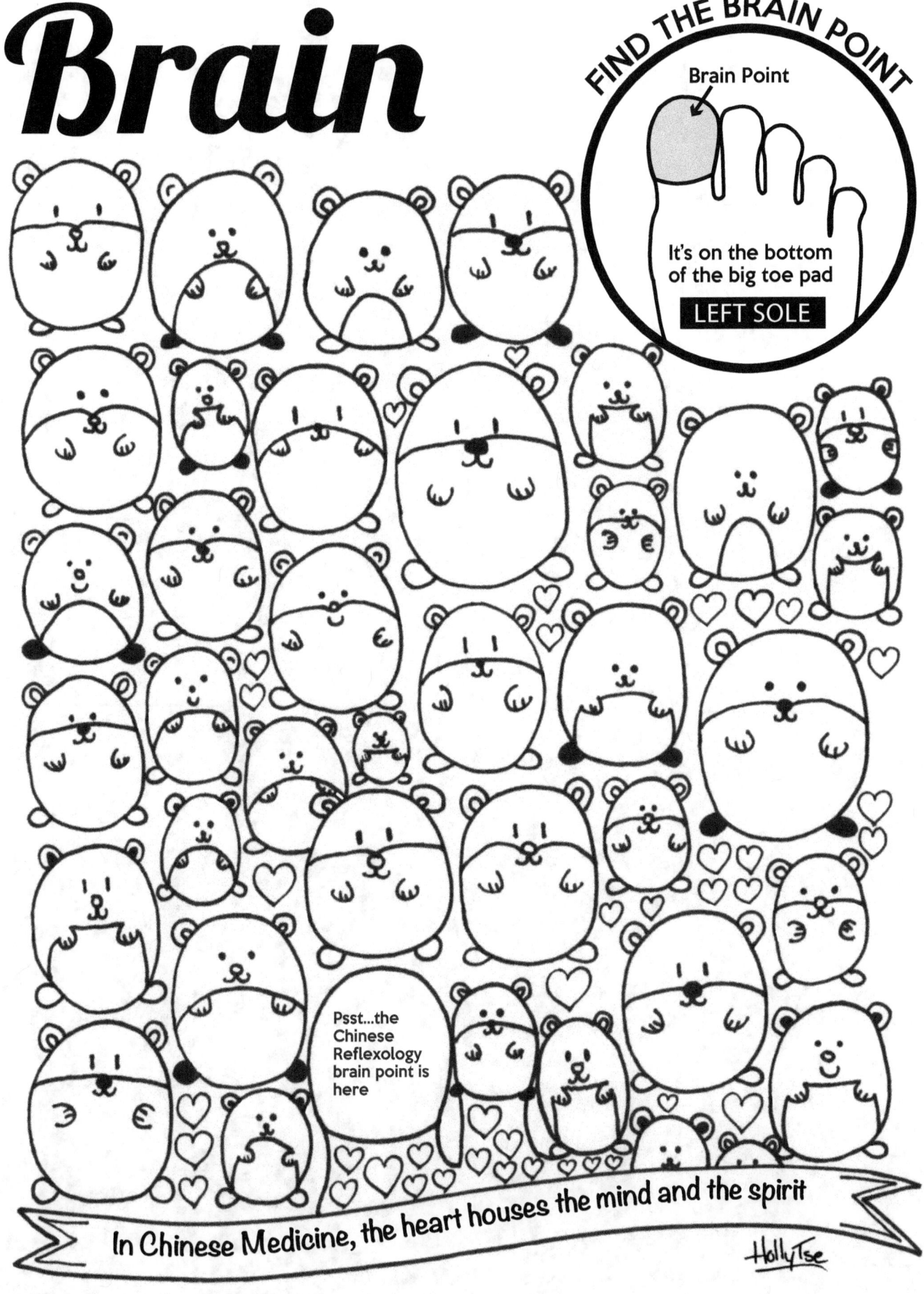

Brain

FIND THE BRAIN POINT

Brain Point

It's on the bottom of the big toe pad

LEFT SOLE

Psst...the Chinese Reflexology brain point is here

In Chinese Medicine, the heart houses the mind and the spirit

HollyTse

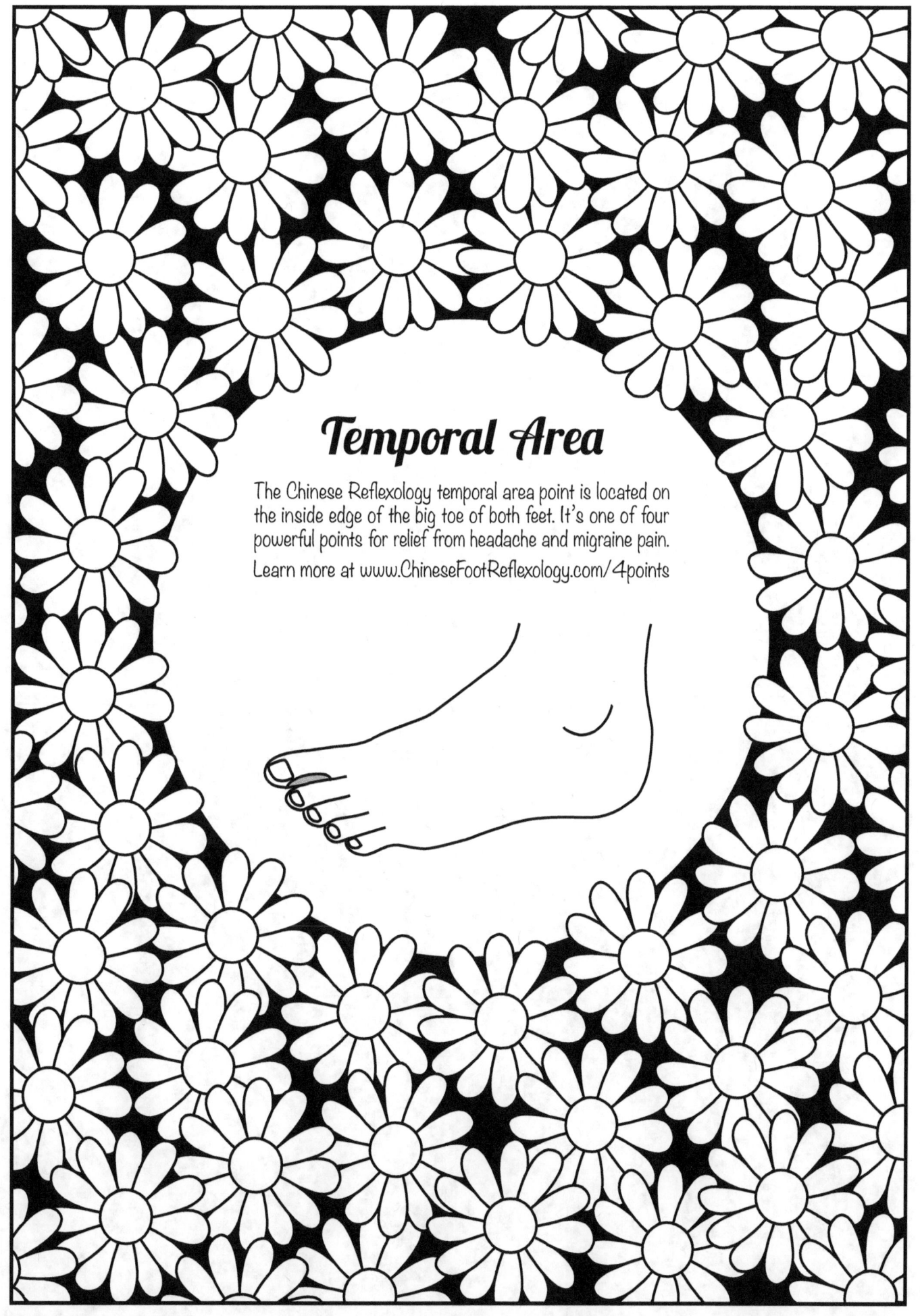

Temporal Area

The Chinese Reflexology temporal area point is located on the inside edge of the big toe of both feet. It's one of four powerful points for relief from headache and migraine pain.

Learn more at www.ChineseFootReflexology.com/4points

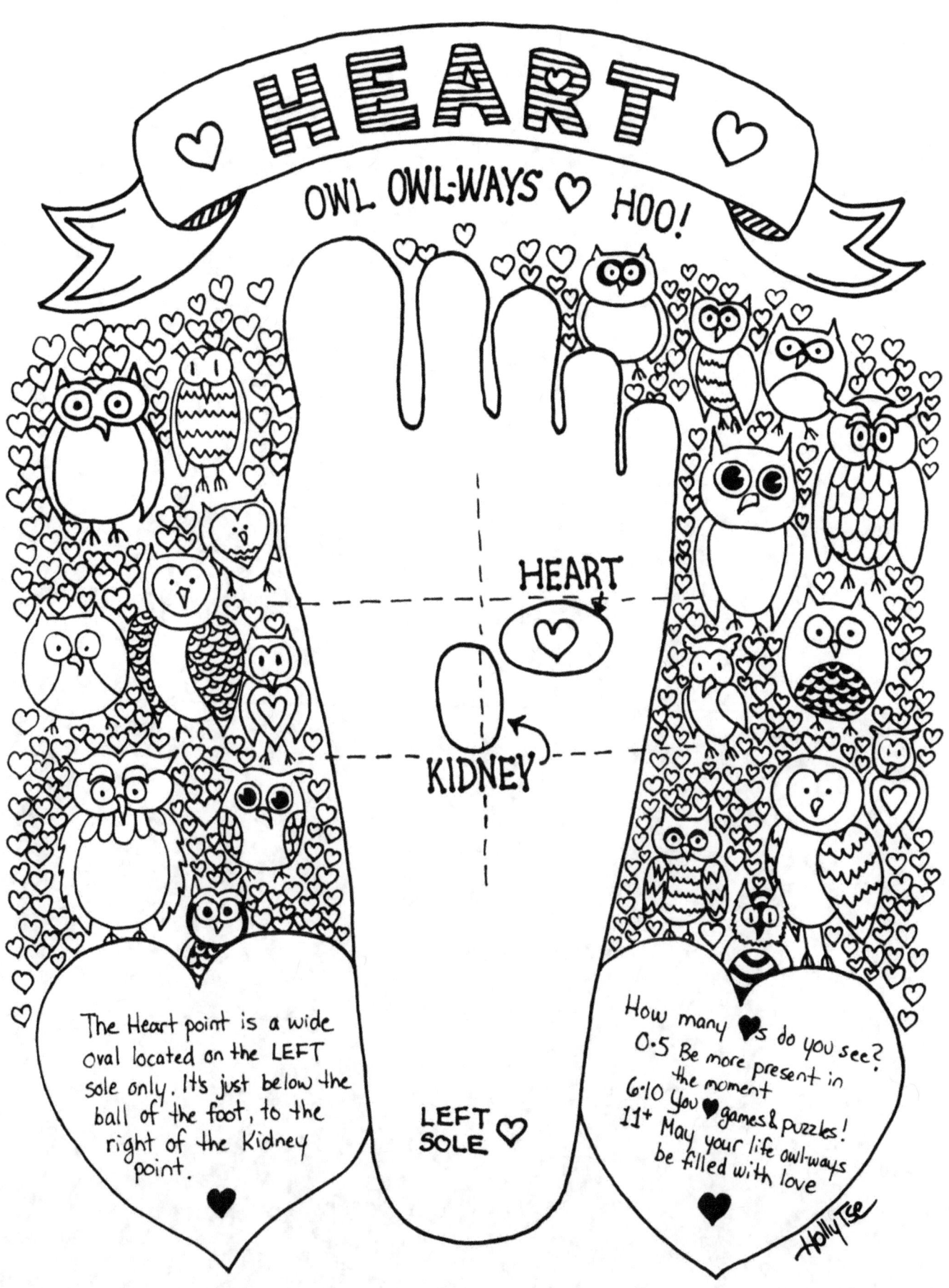

HEART

OWL OWL-WAYS ♡ HOO!

HEART

KIDNEY

LEFT SOLE ♡

The Heart point is a wide oval located on the LEFT sole only. It's just below the ball of the foot, to the right of the Kidney point. ♥

How many ♥s do you see?
0-5 Be more present in the moment
6-10 You ♥ games & puzzles!
11+ May your life owl-ways be filled with love ♥

Holly Tse

Solar Plexus

The Chinese Reflexology solar plexus point is a small circle on the soles of both feet. Imagine a vertical line dividing the foot in half vertically. This point is in a small indent that's on or close to this line, just below the ball of the foot.

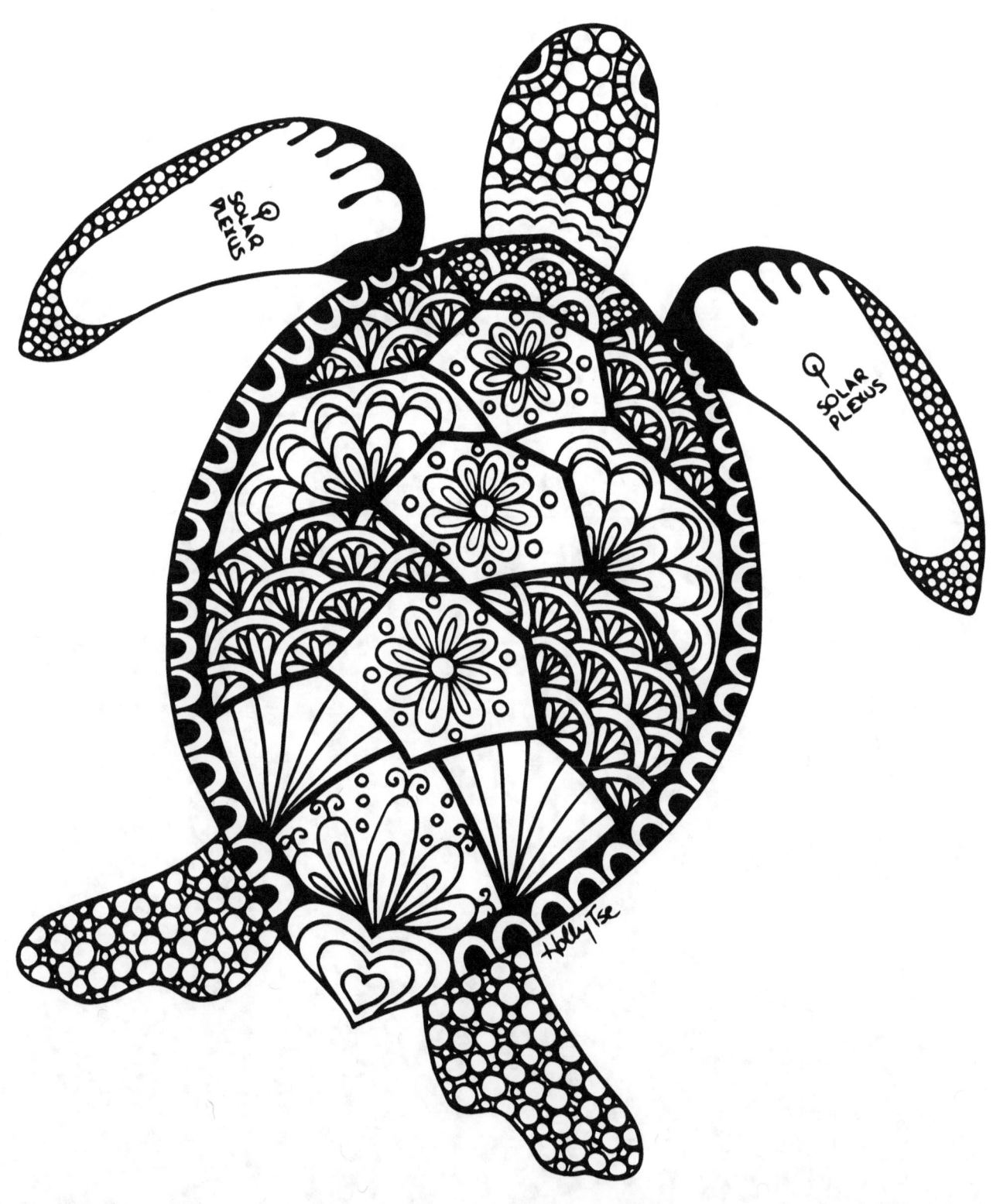

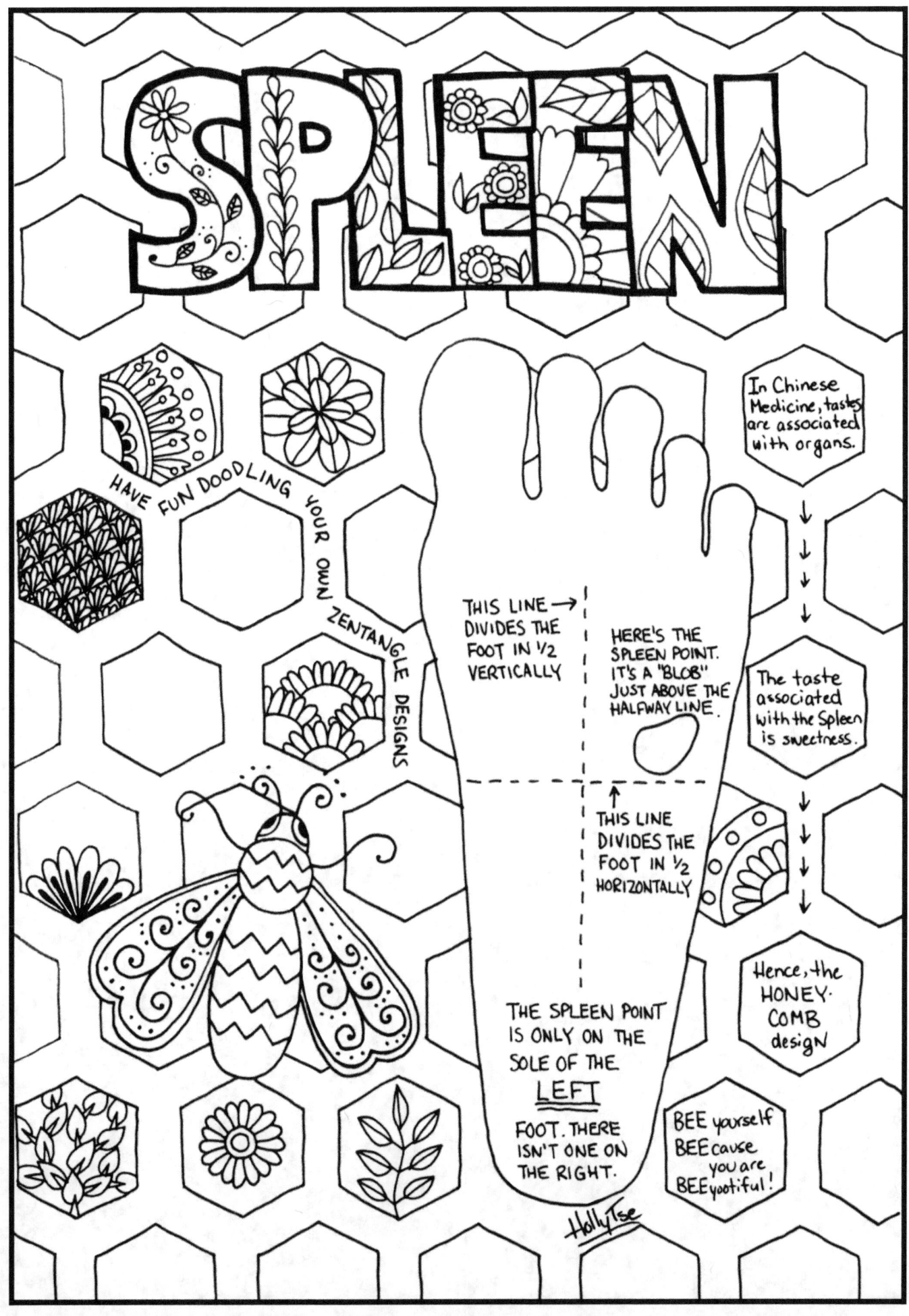

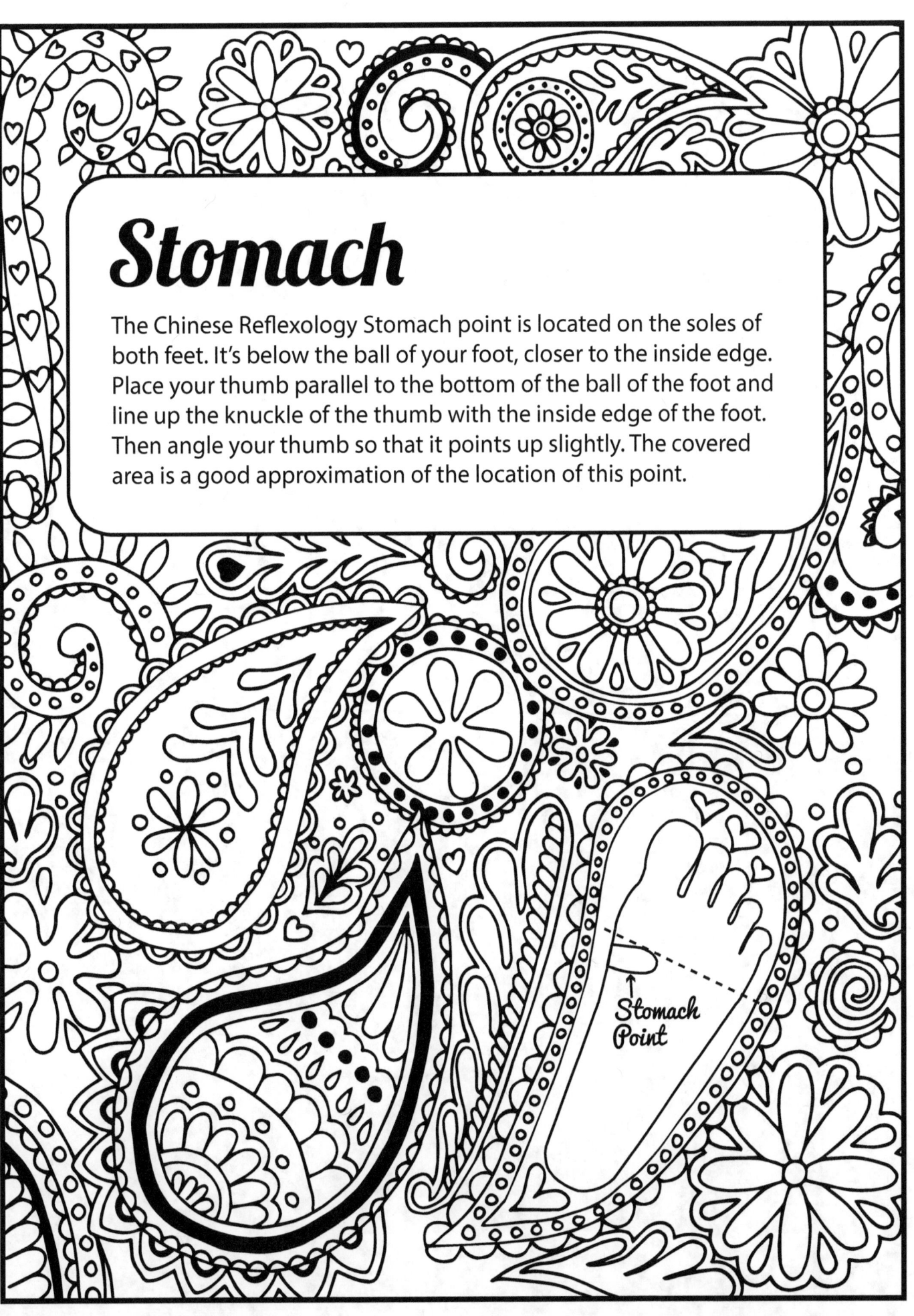

Stomach

The Chinese Reflexology Stomach point is located on the soles of both feet. It's below the ball of your foot, closer to the inside edge. Place your thumb parallel to the bottom of the ball of the foot and line up the knuckle of the thumb with the inside edge of the foot. Then angle your thumb so that it points up slightly. The covered area is a good approximation of the location of this point.

Stomach Point

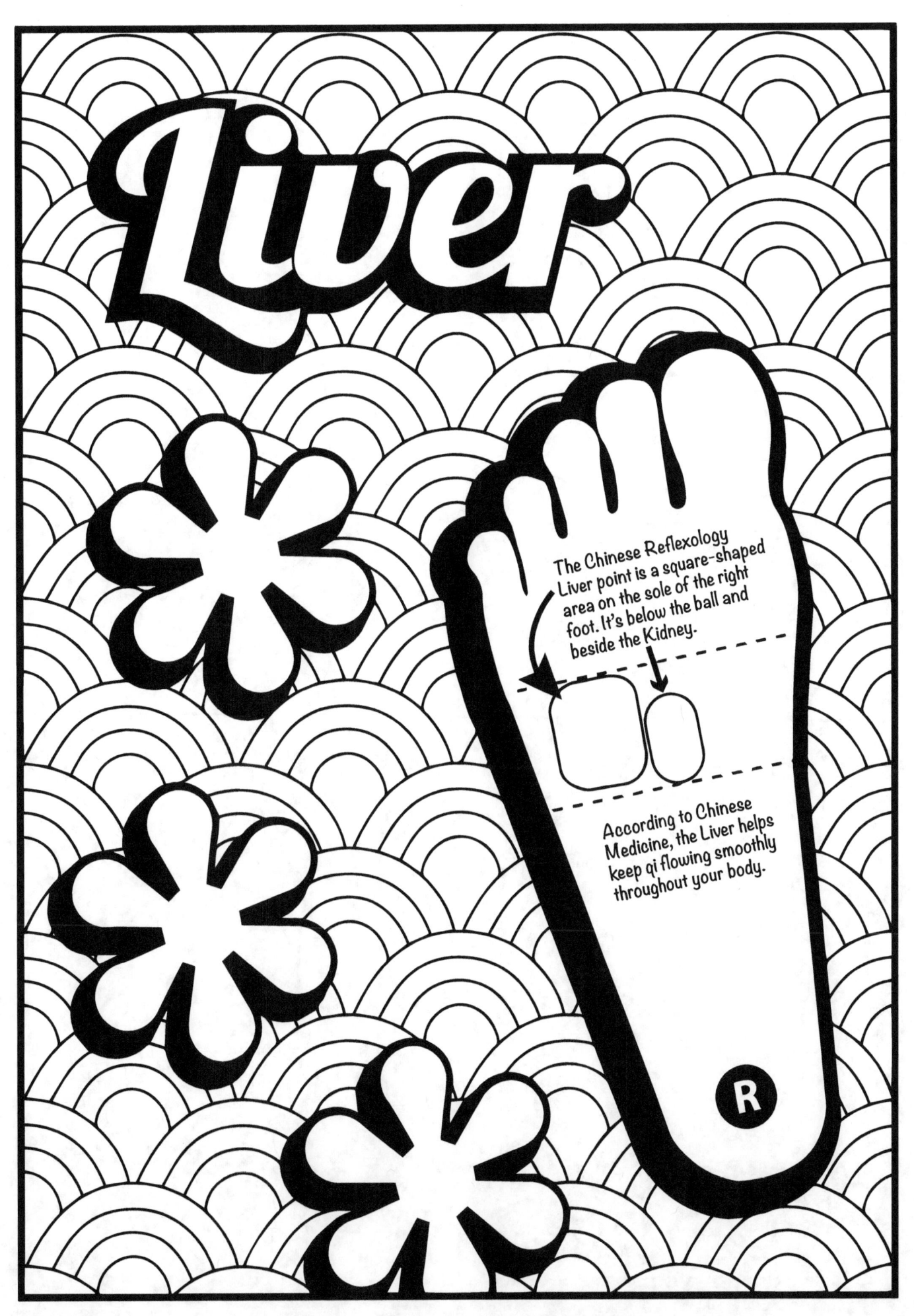

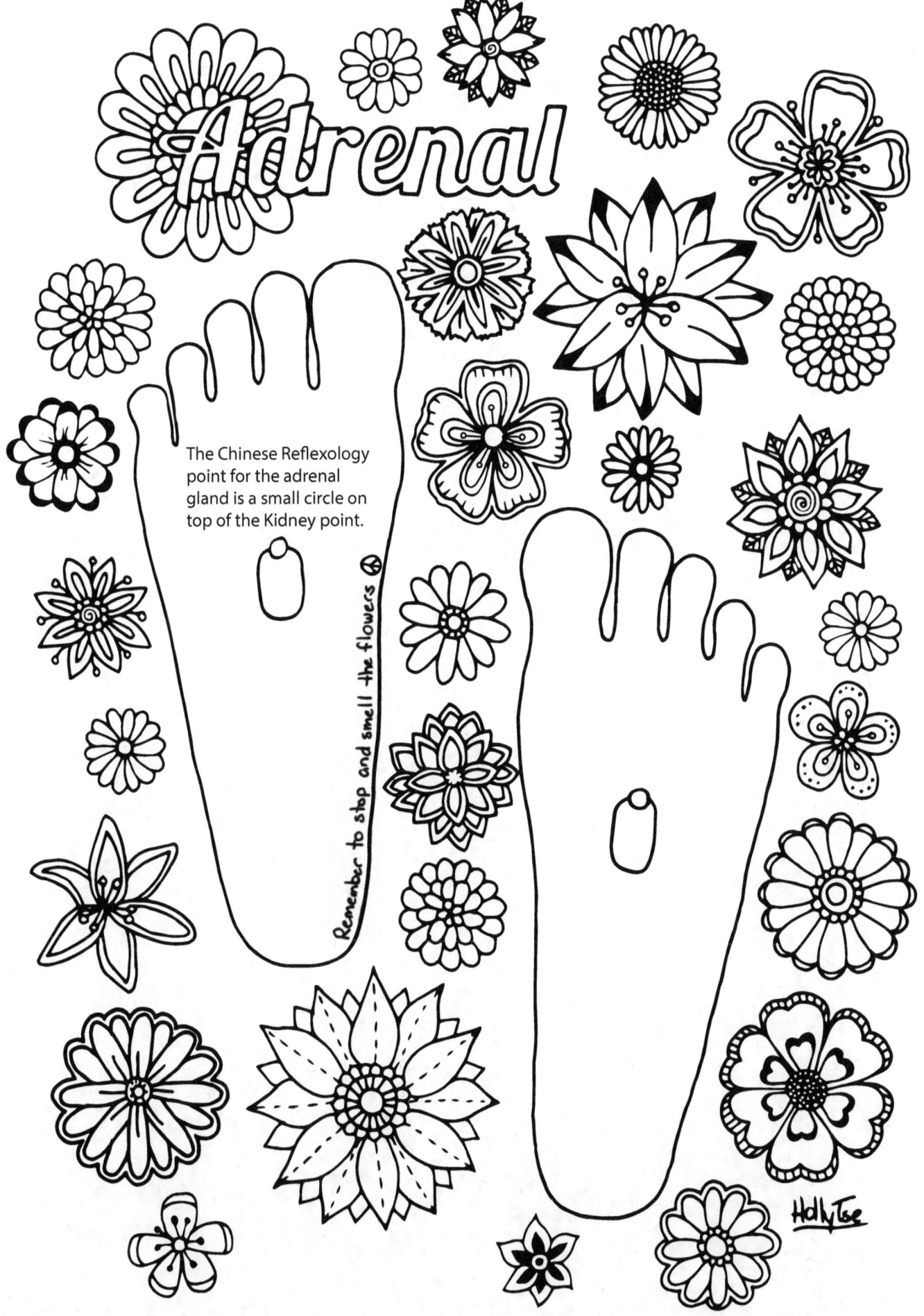

Adrenal

The Chinese Reflexology point for the adrenal gland is a small circle on top of the Kidney point.

Remember to stop and smell the flowers

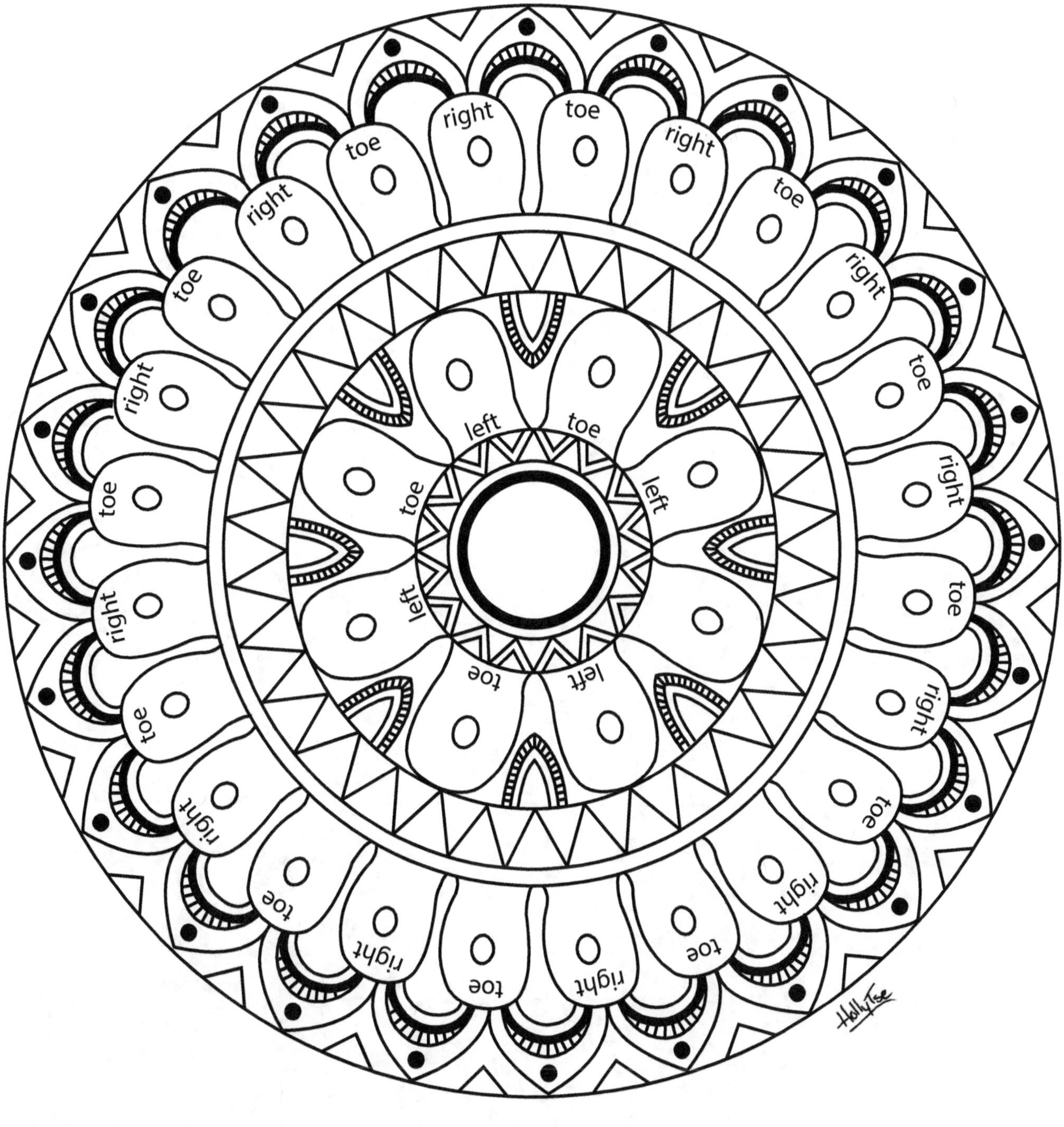

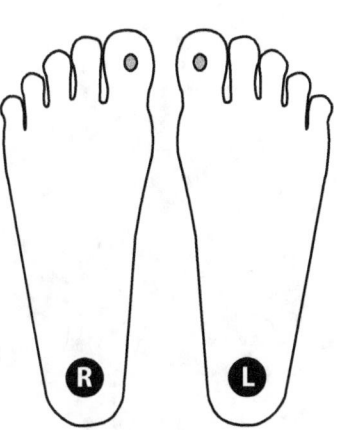

Pituitary Gland

The pituitary gland is often referred to as the master gland because it produces and secretes hormones that influence other endocrine glands. This Chinese Reflexology point is a small circle in the middle of the big toe pad. It's slightly off center, closer to the inside edge of the foot. Coloring in 32 toe pads will help you remember this point!

R   L

Chinese Reflexology Large Intestine Hand Points

These points are looking peacocky
But take care not to be cocky
Don't make a guess
And randomly press
Instead, learn the right thing to do
At ChineseFootReflexology.com/poo

Transverse Colon

Anus

Points are only for the LEFT palm. They follow the flow of qi through the colon.

Sigmoid Colon

Descending Colon

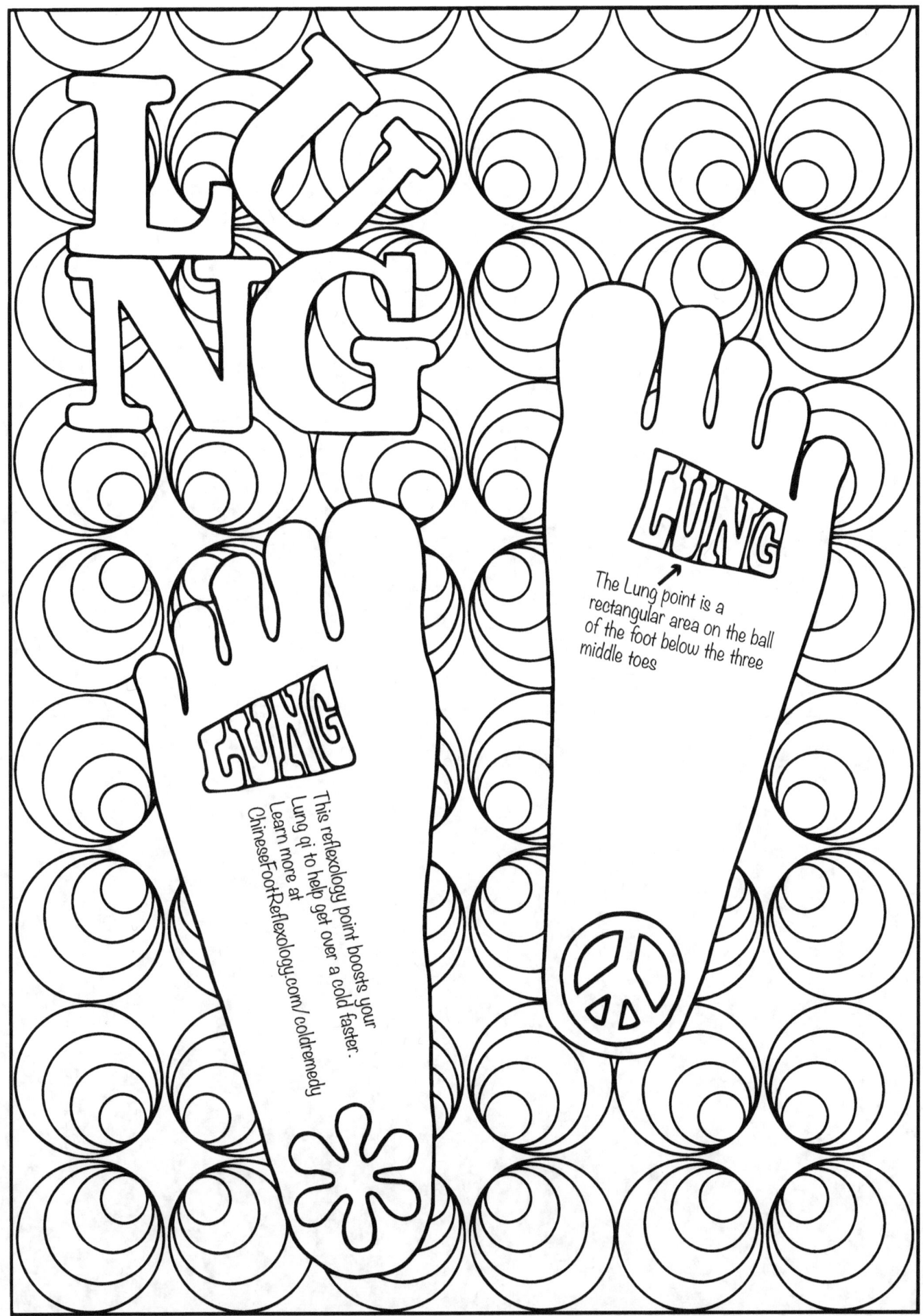

LUNG

LUNG

The Lung point is a rectangular area on the ball of the foot below the three middle toes

LUNG

This reflexology point boosts your Lung qi to help get over a cold faster. Learn more at ChineseFootReflexology.com/coldremedy

Gall Bladder

This Chinese Reflexology point is a small circle that's only on the sole of the right foot. It's in the top right quadrant of the Liver point. Strong Gall Bladder qi is associated with courage and decisiveness. In Chinese Medicine, this organ is spelled as two words.

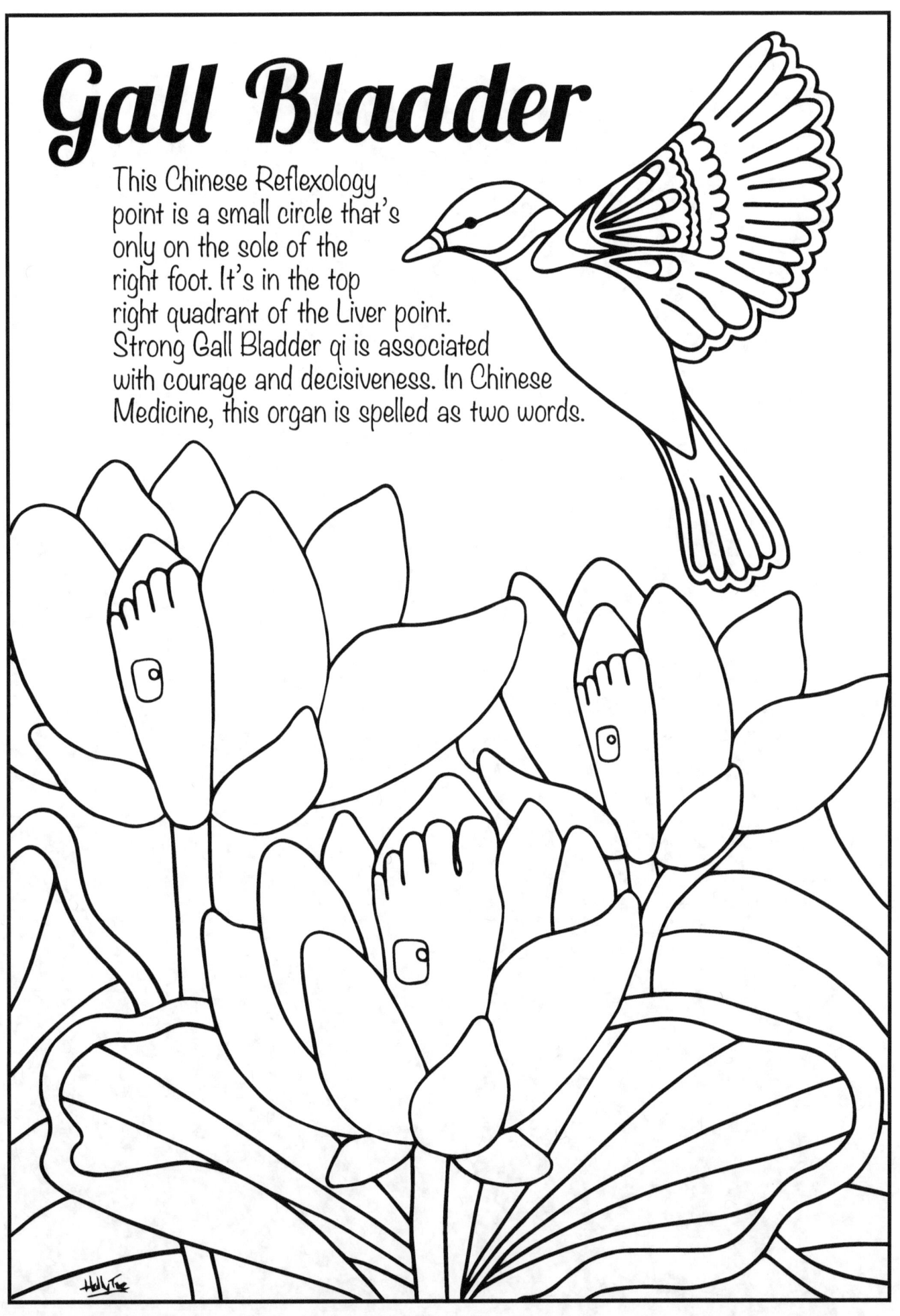

Shoulder Point

The Chinese Reflexology shoulder point is a fleshy rectangular area located on the sole of the foot just below the pinky toe. The right foot is for the right shoulder and the left foot is for the left shoulder.

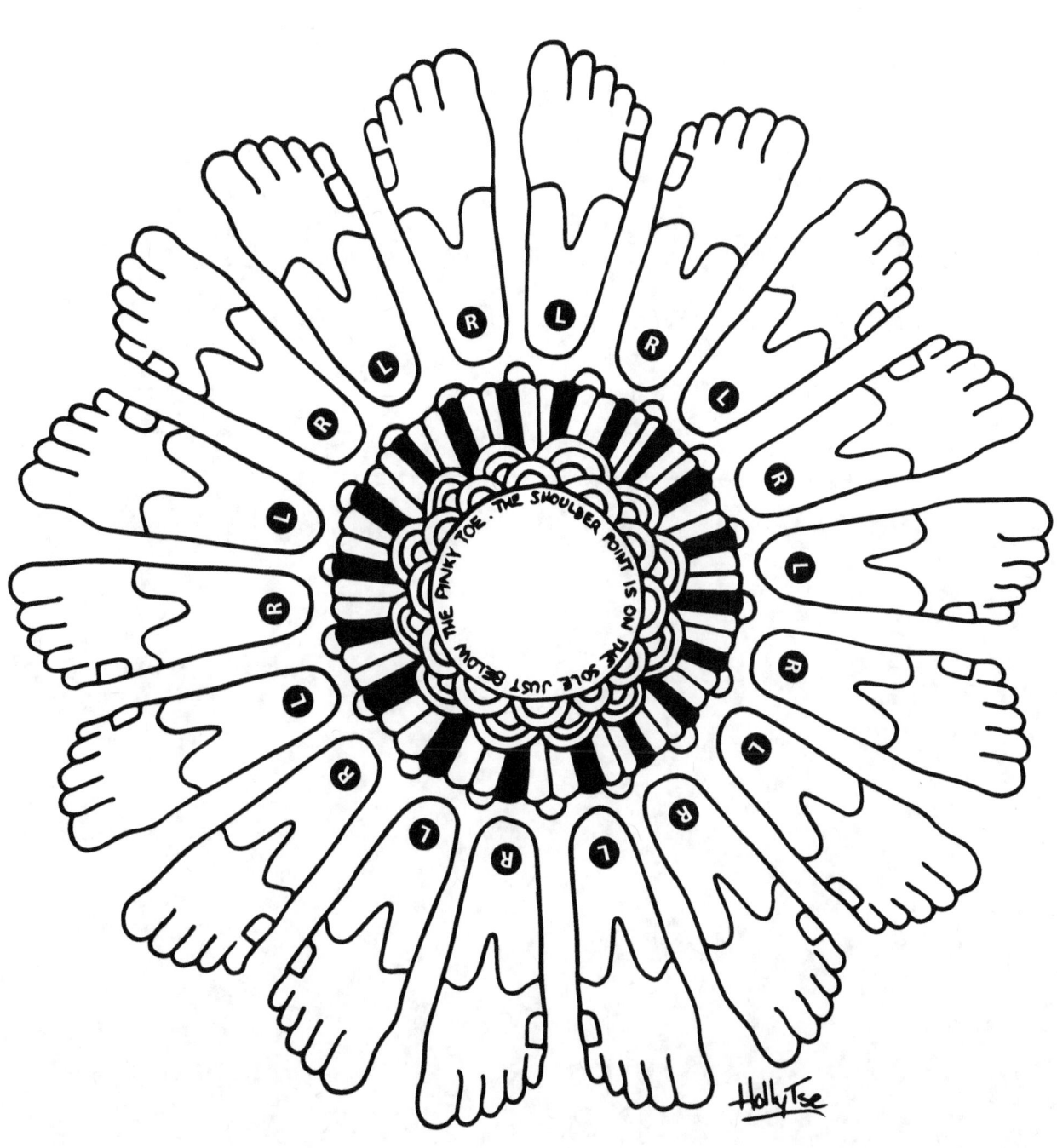

THE SHOULDER POINT IS ON THE SOLE JUST BELOW THE PINKY TOE.

HollyTse

Knee

The Chinese Reflexology knee point is on the outer edge of the foot. It's a semi-circlular area in a small depression in front of the heel, with a diameter slightly wider than the width of your thumb.

KNEE

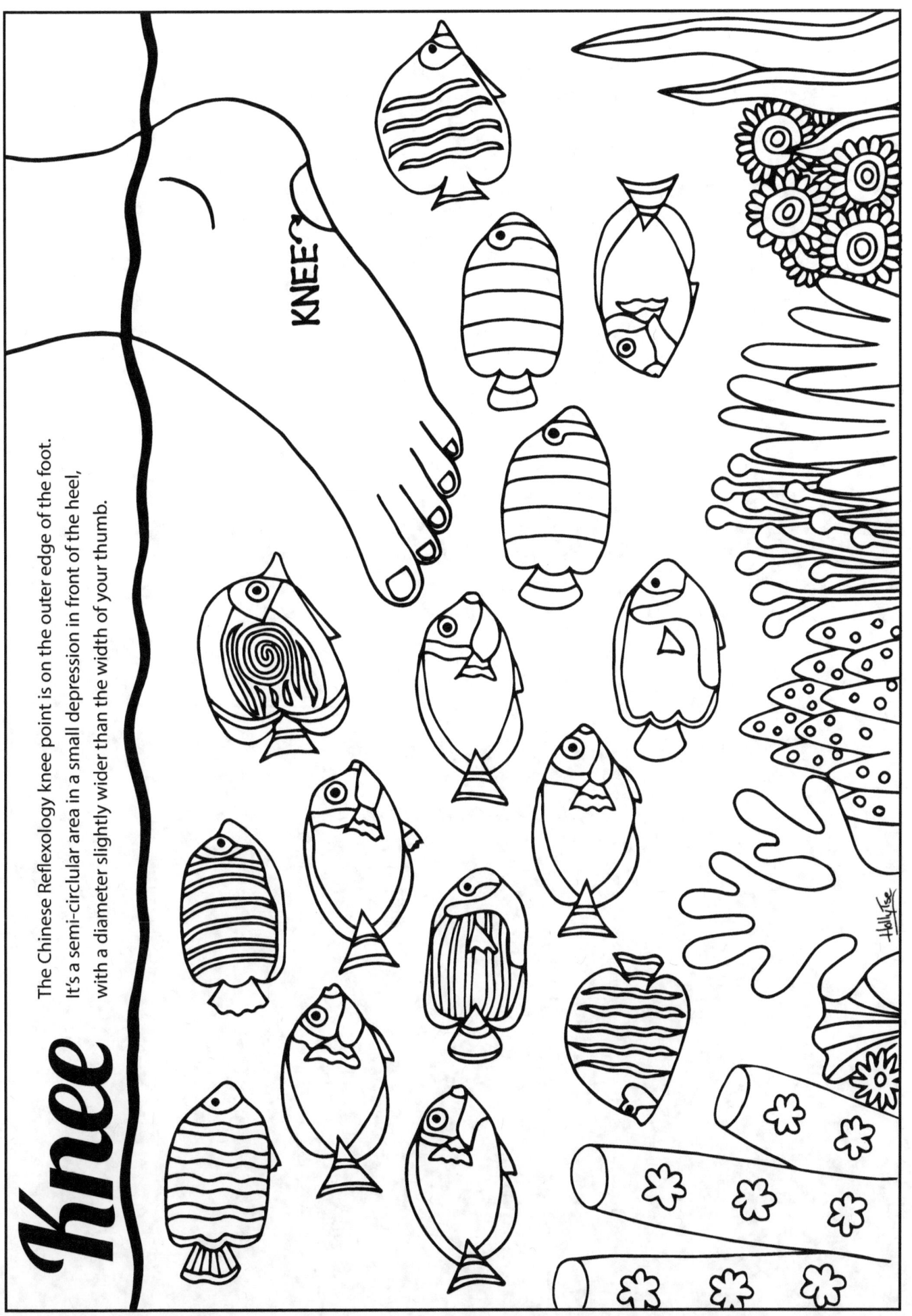

Inner & Outer Hip

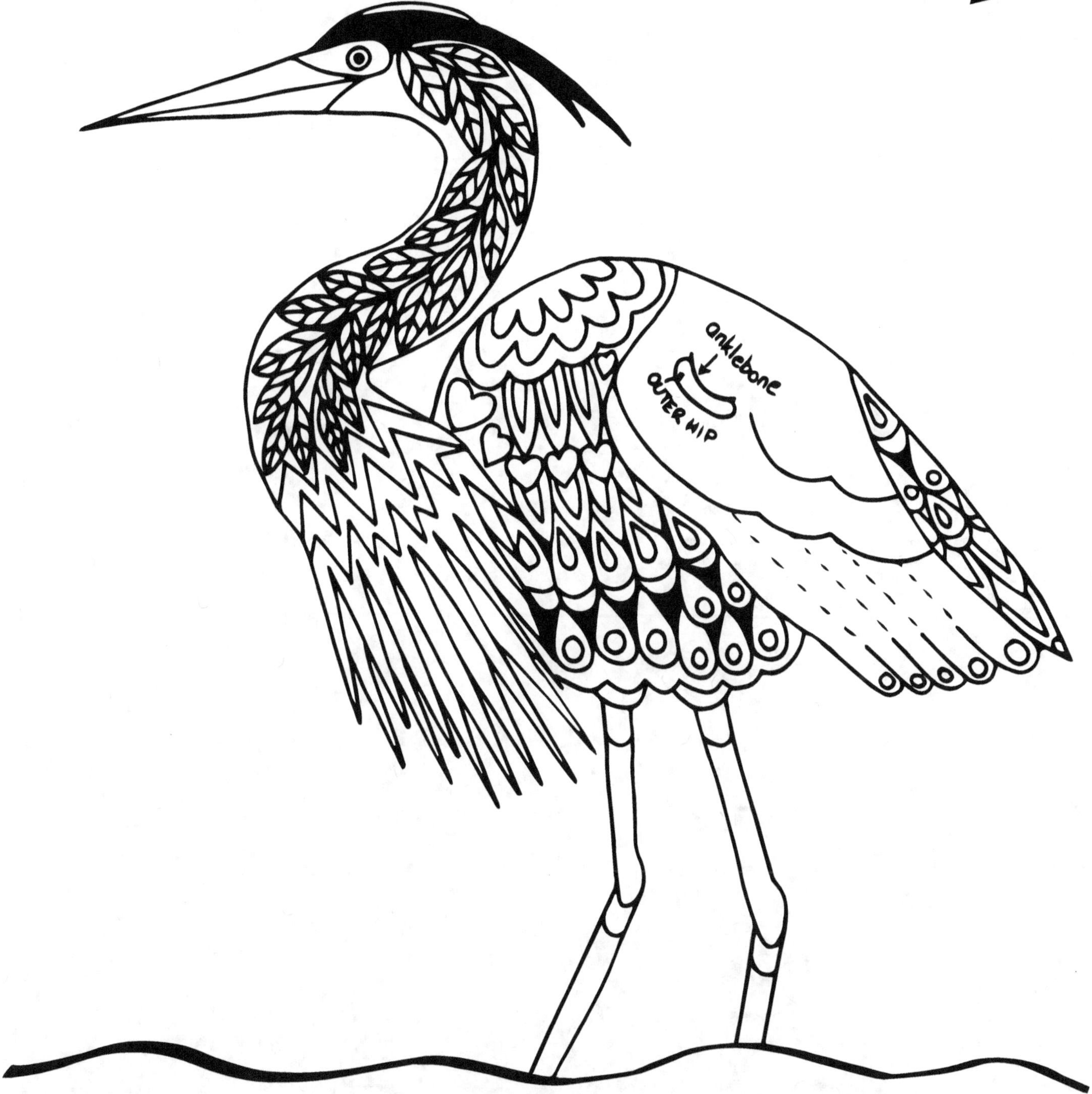

anklebone

OUTER HIP

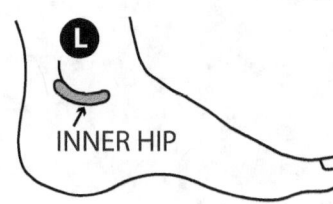

L

INNER HIP

The Chinese Reflexology hip points are tube-shaped areas just below and slightly behind the anklebone. The inside of the ankle is for the inner hip point, and the outside is for the outer hip point. Great Blue Herons can grow up to 4.5 feet high with a 6-foot wingspan.

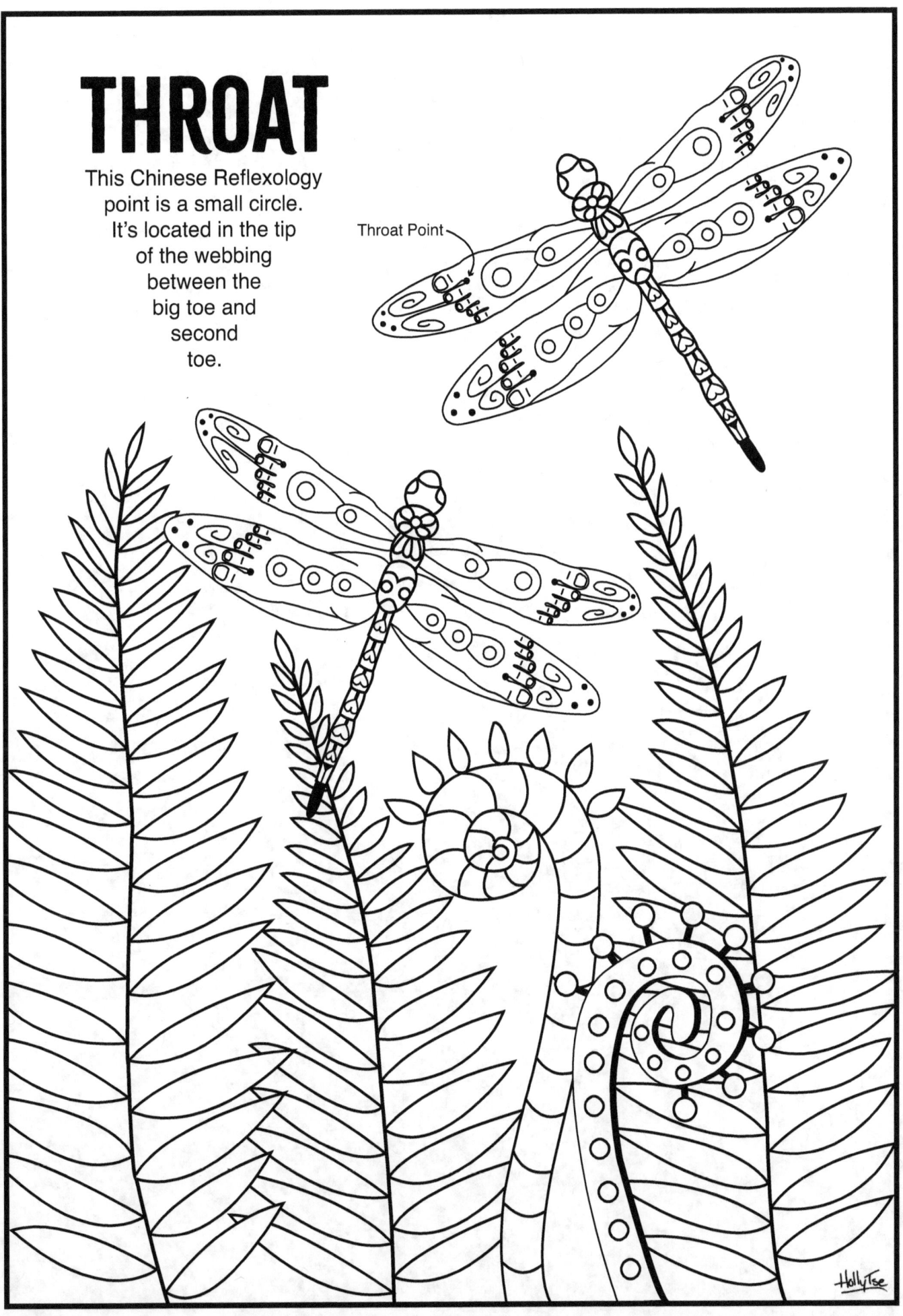

THROAT

This Chinese Reflexology point is a small circle. It's located in the tip of the webbing between the big toe and second toe.

Throat Point

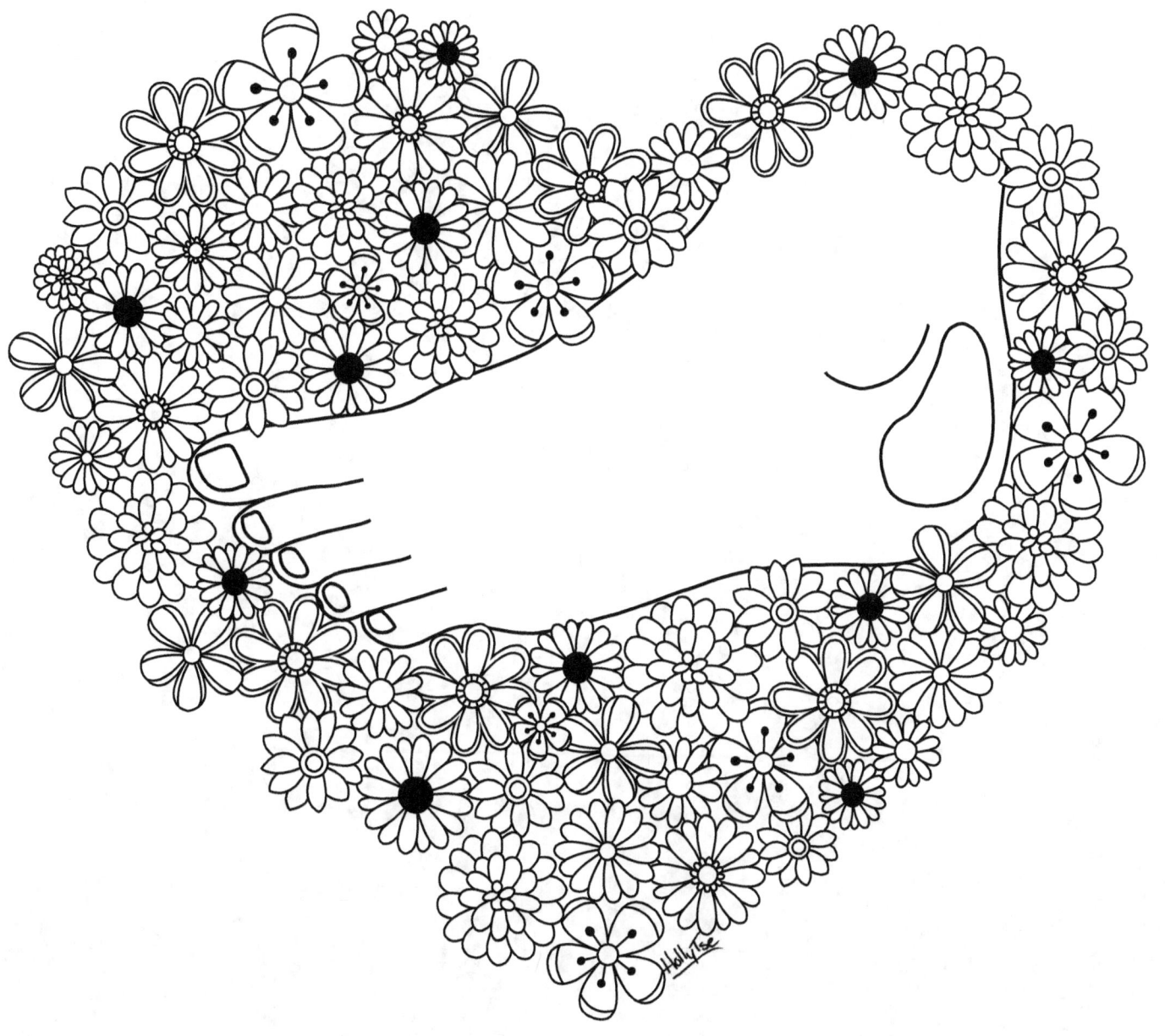

Ovaries & Testicles

This Chinese Reflexology point is a teardrop-shaped area on the outside edge of the foot. It's located just below and behind the anklebone on both the right and left feet. For women, it's the ovary point, and for men, it's the testicle point.

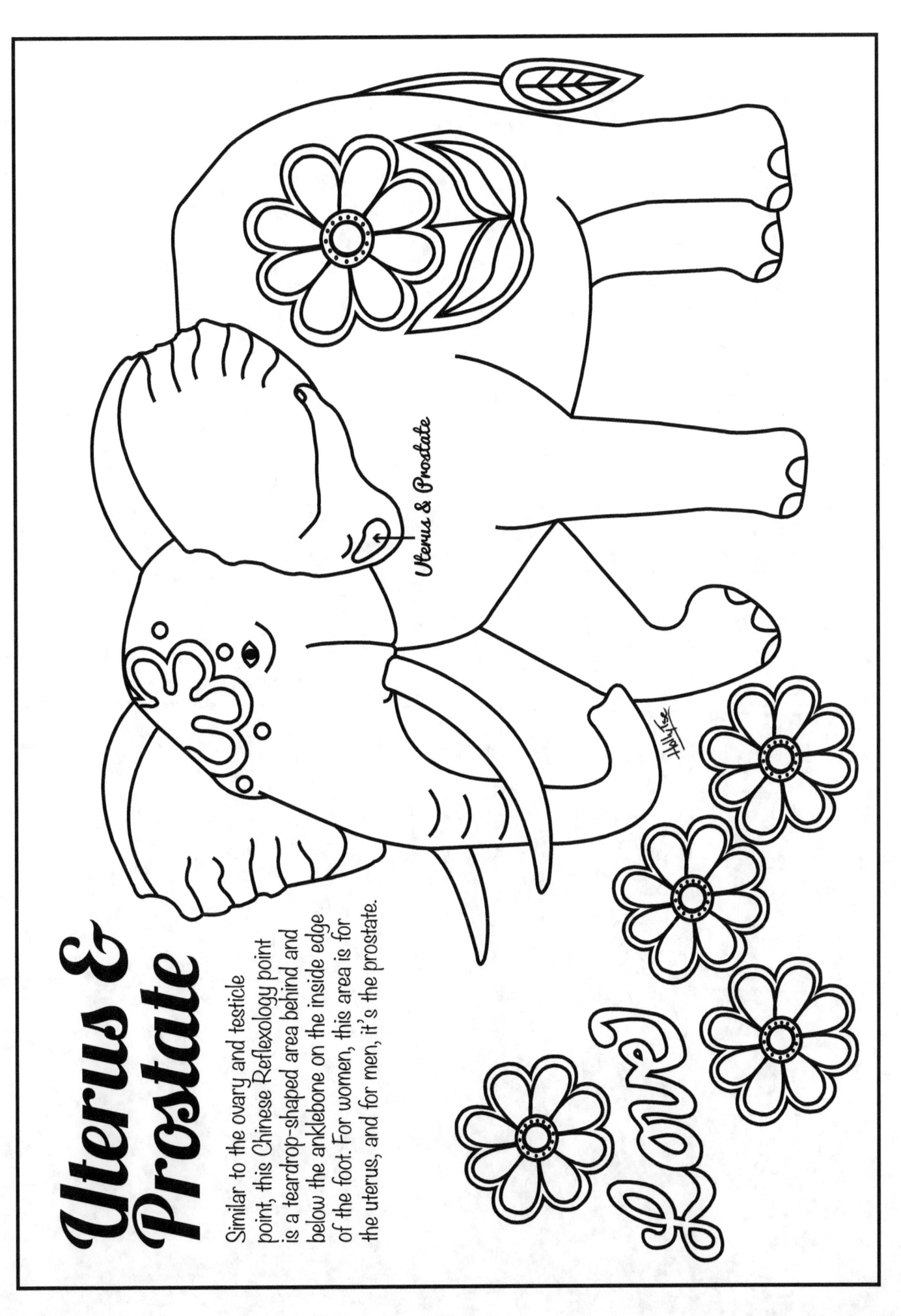

Uterus & Prostate

Similar to the ovary and testicle point, this Chinese Reflexology point is a teardrop-shaped area behind and below the anklebone on the inside edge of the foot. For women, this area is for the uterus, and for men, it's the prostate.

Uterus & Prostate

love

A Page to Test Colors

A Page to Doodle

Create your own doodles and designs here. When you allow your creativity to flow, you'll also get your qi flowing.

3 WAYS TO LEARN MORE

1. Sole Guidance

Learn how to practice Chinese Reflexology at home with Holly's book, *Sole Guidance*. It's a brilliant introduction to this ancient healing art of foot massage. Discover how fun and easy it is to use Chinee Reflexology to improve your health and well-being. ISBN: 978-1401949273

Learn more at: www.ChineseFootReflexology.com/book

2. ChineseFootReflexology.com

Visit Holly's groundbreaking website for an incredible resource of free articles and mini lessons on how to use Chinese Reflexology for a variety of health ailments, including cold recovery and prevention, headache and migraine relief, knee pain, breast health, and more. Sign up for Holly's complimentary monthly newsletter for free lessons, quick reference charts, special events and more.

Get the free newsletter and lessons at: www.ChineseFootReflexology.com

3. Sole Fundamentals & Sole Mastery

Learn Chinese Reflexology with Holly as your teacher. Holly teaches two online programs, each taught once per year. Sole Fundamentals is her 6-week introductory course to Chinese Reflexology, and Sole Mastery is her in depth 6-month program to help you be in command of your health and destiny. Join the waitlist for special early bird registration savings and to be notified of the next session. Holly also offers special workshops on different topics throughout the year.

Join the waitlist for savings at: www.ChineseFootReflexology.com/workshops

ABOUT THE AUTHOR & ILLUSTRATOR

Holly Tse is the founder of ChineseFootReflexology.com, the premier English language website on Chinese Reflexology, with readers from over 200 countries worldwide. She is also the author of the internationally bestselling book, *Sole Guidance: Ancient Secrets of Chinese Reflexology to Heal the Body, Mind, Heart, and Spirit*.

Holly illustrated all of the coloring pages in this book. She used a combination of computer design and inking by hand. When she's not doodling, you'll find her hiking, swimming, biking or spoiling her 18-year old cat.

www.ingramcontent.com/pod-product-compliance
Lightning Source LLC
Chambersburg PA
CBHW052010280526
45793CB00005B/922